COVID CANCER
CRAIC

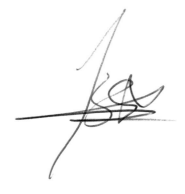

Published under licence by Brown Dog Books and
The Self-Publishing Partnership Ltd, 10b Greenway Farm, Bath Rd,
Wick, nr. Bath BS30 5RL

www.selfpublishingpartnership.co.uk

ISBN printed book: 978-1-83952-423-3
ISBN e-book: 978-1-83952-424-0

Cover design by Andrew Prescott
Internal design by Andrew Easton

Printed and bound in the UK

This book is printed on FSC certified paper

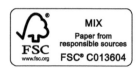

COVID CANCER CRAIC

Coping with a death sentence through memories and laughter

Issy Hogg

BROWN
DOG
BOOKS

Acknowledgements

Particular thanks go to my sisters, Philippa Watt and Kate Fleming, for being there.

I would also like to thank all of my friends on my Odyssey page for taking the time to read my musings. Your comments and support have been so uplifting and encouraging. I would especially like to thank Sue Cooper, Clare Mortimer, Issy Bramah and Chris Hanson for reading this book in draft form and providing such helpful feedback.

I am extremely grateful to Wayne Barnes, internationally renowned rugby union referee, respected barrister and Breast Cancer Now ambassador for taking a very supportive interest in my story and kindly providing the foreword.

Additional thanks go to Douglas Walker and Frances Prior-Reeves at the Self-Publishing Partnership for helping to turn my ambition into reality.

*To Vic and Leah for selflessly providing me with
endless love and support*

*To The Thin Controller (aka Dr Marcus Remer)
and his team at the Shunting Shed (aka the Rainbow
Unit at Basingstoke Hospital).
Thank you for extending my gift of life.*

Foreword

This book is not only a great thing because it supports an essential charity – Breast Cancer Now – but it also offers you a look into the mind of a person who's been confronted with some of the worst news you can possibly receive, and has her own unique way of dealing with it. Issy doesn't just tell her story, but she also demonstrates her belief that a positive mindset and upbeat approach secures the most beneficial response to treatment for those living with cancer, in addition to the best outcomes in life.

Issy's outlook resonates hugely with me, and there's food for thought inside these pages no matter where you are in life, and whatever your challenges.

My wife, Polly, lost her Mum to breast cancer. Debbie Broderick was only 56 years old. In the UK a woman dies from breast cancer every 45 minutes and is the leading cause of death in women under 50. When you let that sink in, you see how it touches every one of us in some way.

But because of the amazing work of charities like Breast Cancer Now, almost nine in ten women survive breast cancer for five years or more, with survival rates having doubled in the past 40 years.

Each year, Polly and I hold an annual rugby event in Polly's mum's honour, in support of Breast Cancer Now. That is our little part in supporting a wonderful cause. This is Issy's.

Wayne Barnes

Contents

I

Raison d'Être

Being diagnosed with Stage 4 metastatic breast cancer, spreading extensively through my bones, showing up in my liver and lungs and with a life-expectancy prognosis of six months, was not how I imagined a Covid-19 pandemic lockdown would commence in March 2020. The fact that I had fought off breast cancer sixteen years previously, and been given the all-clear after tailored Zoladex and Tamoxifen treatment, made the news even more difficult to comprehend.

The sudden and dramatic change to my previously calm and well-ordered world included an initial nine-day period of hospitalisation that coincided with the commencement of lockdown and an associated ban on visiting time. This was followed by long-term shielding at home with my husband, Vic, necessitated by my vulnerability arising from the start of chemotherapy treatment and the fractures to my neck (requiring a permanent neck brace) and ribs caused by the spread of cancer.

The extent of my vulnerability also meant evacuating my daughter, Leah, and pet dog, Harvey, to close friends five miles away in Alton, Hampshire, and ceasing visits to my then ninety-one-year-old mother who was residing in a nearby nursing home due to her dementia.

My condition also meant the loss of a degree of independence, including the ability to drive, and spelled the end of my long, successful and fulfilling legal career.

But I was determined to adapt to these enforced changes and not be dispirited by the hand I had been dealt. I focused on remaining positive and upbeat and continuing to enjoy life to the full. I set up a closed Facebook page with the intention of keeping family and friends updated with my progress. I named it *Issy's Odyssey*.

In no time at all I found myself posting on a daily basis – reflecting on my past life, providing insights into my legal career, sharing my interest in various hobbies and pastimes, ranting about current news events, as well as updating on medical progress. I found my daily efforts to be enjoyable and cathartic. My musings helped to maintain my positivity.

To my delight the posts were well received, with friends telling me that they had become essential daily reading. I was humbled to be told that I was inspirational. It was not long before I was being encouraged to turn my musings into print. Hence this book was born.

This is not intended to be an autobiography. After all, I am not a celebrity, not even a D-lister. It is a record of my journey through treatment thus far, peppered with some light-hearted anecdotes. I regard myself as extremely lucky in possessing natural *joie de vivre* – my glass is always half full (except where Pinot Grigio is involved and allowed!). I am very strongly of the belief that a positive mindset and upbeat approach represent key elements in securing the best outcomes in life, including the most beneficial response to treatment for those living with cancer. I am determined to spread this message as far as I possibly can, using my own experiences as persuasive evidence.

In so doing I would regard it as a major triumph if my story also encourages a positive approach to cancer and cancer treatment in those who perceive only fear and dread based on historic misconceptions and the predominantly negative press that the disease attracts.

2

A Cancer Calls

My first brush with the Big C was in June 2004. I was two months shy of my forty-fourth birthday and my daughter, Leah, had just turned seven. As with the recurrence in 2020, the initial diagnosis of breast cancer came out of the blue, a complete shock.

I had been jumping on Leah's trampoline, a pastime that I am sure many adults have taken part in while enjoying a convivial summer party with friends in the garden! The following day I noticed that my right breast appeared a little misshapen. It just so happened that my husband, Vic (who, for reasons that will be explained later, will from now on be referred to as Vinny) and I already had routine appointments booked at the Hampshire Clinic in Old Basing for personal MOTs and mine included a Well Woman check.

On attending that check and being examined, my planned mammogram was immediately cancelled and an appointment made for me to see a consultant a few days later.

That appointment was a surreal experience. Although I was stunned by the diagnosis when formally delivered, in reality Vinny and I knew beforehand, in our heart of hearts, that something was not quite right. We pretended all was well and attended the appointment both dressed in suits, with the intention of going to work immediately afterwards. We had, however, driven there in total silence – unusual for us, but clearly indicative of our anxious states of mind.

Within nine days of the diagnosis, I found myself an inpatient at the Hampshire Clinic, undergoing a mastectomy and a latissimus-dorsi reconstruction.

In the time between diagnosis and hospital admission, I believed that I was functioning perfectly normally. Being a criminal defence solicitor, I continued to attend courts and police stations in the usual way but my then secretary subsequently told me that my dictation was utter garbage. I would start a letter, tail off in the middle and start another.

At home I went into a form of overdrive. I filled the freezer with home-cooked meals for Vinny and Leah, along with writing out a detailed log of Leah's daily school activities and uniform requirements. Fortunately, Leah was just a little too young to understand what was happening but I wanted Vinny's time, while I was in hospital, to be as stress-free as possible. I knew it would be difficult for him, not least because his mother died of breast cancer when he was only five years old and the hospital visits remain one of his few memories of her.

Thankfully, by the time of my admission to the Hampshire Clinic, I had had a serious word with myself and had fully accepted the diagnosis. I was very positive and upbeat about the procedure, actually laughing my way through the eight days I spent there. Because I was always cheerful, people were happy to chat with me. Consequently, I had a constant stream of visitors and my room looked like a florist's shop. That, in turn, made my stay much more bearable. I insisted on having my door open as I did not want to feel shut away.

Vinny and Leah visited daily and often had a meal with me despite all my efforts waiting for them at home in the freezer. Vinny was even provided with a beer or two. The nurses were always popping in for a chinwag and started their morning drug rounds with me.

The mastectomy and latissimus-dorsi reconstruction were performed within the same five-hour operation by two consultants – one for the mastectomy and the other for the reconstruction. For the uninitiated, as I was then, the latissimus dorsi is the large muscle across the back and, in my case, was used to help in reconstructing my breast following the mastectomy, hence the name of the procedure. When Vinny placed the name of the operation into a spellcheck for the purposes of an insurance claim, it came out as "luscious doris". Since then, my right breast has been known as Luscious Doris. I reported this to my consultant who looked at me as though I had become unhinged!

On the morning after the operation, I was still not quite with it, so did not question the nature of medication supplied to me. It was not long before the walls started moving in and out as if the air was being sucked from the room and then pumped back in again. I had been given Tramadol, a strong painkiller often used after surgery. Knowing of its potential to cause addiction, and not wanting to experience such weird side effects again, I declined any further doses and survived on paracetamol.

As well as being entertained by my visitors, there were some amusing incidents involving other patients. On one occasion the man in the next room to me returned from theatre suffering from a reaction to the anaesthetic. During the night I heard him talking to Huey on the great white porcelain telephone. When I enquired the following morning after his welfare, the deputy matron gave him short shrift by saying, "Well, he's a man isn't he!" What more could you say?

On another occasion Paddy arrived from Ireland on the back of his mate's motorbike. It was a Sunday afternoon. Having checked in, the pair of them sneaked out to the pub. The ward was run by a fearsome matron with whom I actually got on very well. On the return of the likely lads from the pub, I heard Matron say in her best Lady Bracknell voice, "You've had *how* many?" I cheekily queried with Matron whether Paddy would be able to have his operation. She said it would depend on his state the next morning. I never did find out what happened to him. Good luck if you are ever a man in hospital showing the slightest sign of intolerance to pain or procedure.

Following successful surgery, including removal of the lymph glands under my right arm, I thought of myself as very lucky. The tumour had been in the milk sac, which had acted like cling film. Post-operative histology showed no evidence of cancer cells having escaped into the rest of my body. I did not have any radiotherapy or chemotherapy. I was back at work full-time after eight weeks.

For the next two years I was treated by way of depot injections of Zoladex in my abdomen every twenty-eight days, alongside daily Tamoxifen tablets, which continued for five years. Thereafter I was given the all-clear and, while my brush had caused me to adopt the mindset of ensuring I made the most of life, I thought no more of the Big C.

That was until March 2020.

The year prior to my belated diagnosis in 2020 was, given what I now know about my prevailing condition, quite remarkable.

In April 2019 we flew to the USA, spending a couple of nights in Memphis, Tennessee, before sailing on a paddle steamer down the Mississippi to New Orleans, a trip that had always been on my bucket list.

While in Memphis we were fortunate enough to be able to stay in the Peabody Hotel, home to the internationally famous Peabody Ducks. In the 1930s the general manager at the time had just returned from a weekend shooting and found it amusing to leave his live ducks to play in the hotel fountain, much to the entertainment of the guests. Since then, ducks have spent time in the fountain every day. The hotel employs a duckmaster who, each morning and evening, escorts the ducks to and from their penthouse rooftop quarters via the lift and a red carpet across the lobby to the fountain. It is a delightful spectacle to witness if, at the same time, somewhat ridiculous.

We clearly could not visit Memphis without viewing Graceland. The site is vast, split on either side of a highway with the mansion and grounds on one side and the museums on the other. The latter are well constructed and organised, taking you through various Elvis collections, including musical instruments, awards, outfits, photographs, cars, motorbikes and aeroplanes. The whole collection evokes a strong sense of ostentatiousness and not necessarily all in "the best possible taste".

In contrast, the Graceland mansion is much smaller than we anticipated and had a genuine homely feel to it, albeit spoiled, in our view, by extravagant theming in certain rooms – the Jungle Room, for example, which hopefully speaks for itself! All rooms and grounds were open to the public, including a view of the modest swimming pool, the room where Elvis died and his grave.

Although I grew up more with musicians influenced by Elvis rather than the King himself, I shall never forget the day he died because it was on my seventeenth birthday!

Another iconic building in Memphis is the Lorraine Hotel where Martin Luther King Junior was assassinated. It is now part of the National Civil Rights Museum, a fascinating and informative tribute, even if it does rather macabrely display the actual murder weapon and a recreation of the bathroom from which it was fired.

Following our stay in Memphis we boarded the American Duchess for our leisurely sail through Tennessee and Mississippi to New Orleans in Louisiana. The journey was a fantastic experience, even though it did not quite evoke life as lived by a Mark Twain character, nor present the magnificent river as other than an enormous industrial thoroughfare. (The smell of the oil refinery pollution outside Baton Rouge will long live in my nostrils!). But we visited many historic towns and sites *en route*, from which we learned a great deal about southern music, the American Civil War, civil liberties and the impact of slavery.

At a somewhat different level, life on board the paddle steamer was also an education. Alongside a couple from the West Midlands, we were the only Brits – the rest of the passenger list consisted of septua- and octogenarian American Trump supporters. This worked mainly to our advantage in that we were invariably first to embark and disembark, and take first dibs of every other service and facility on board – apart from the loos, of course!

The demographic also made for interesting conversation at dinner time, with Vinny and I always electing to dine with other couples selected at random to maximise the richness of the overall experience!

As a result, we met potato farmers from North of Seattle, political analysts from New York, golden wedding celebrants from Cleveland (who had not previously been outside Ohio) and a whole host of diverse and interesting characters. The conversations took many unexpected twists and turns. For example, we had dinner one evening with a diplomat's widow from Las Vegas and her gregarious niece from Albuquerque, who had never been outside New Mexico. The latter's conversation was littered with a series of *OMG*s and *Wow*s. We particularly liked the widow's story about how she and her late husband were on the verge of buying Liberace's house following his death – and the couple's rationale for pulling out at the eleventh hour. Evidently, they learned much later than the rest of the world that Liberace had died of an AIDS-related illness. At that point they decided that they could not afford the extensive costs involved in having to fumigate the house before moving in. Nothing we said could dissuade her that such actions and costs would have been completely unnecessary.

I must admit the trip did become a bit of an observation of the quaint habits and utterances of our American brethren. One area that provided much entertainment (and occasional frustration!) was observing their behaviour while on excursions, and the conduct of tour guides.

The paddle steamer was accompanied by two road buses. Each day the vessel moored up at a typical southern antebellum town where the buses were waiting. One of them provided a hop-on, hop-off service. This was ideal for us as it enabled us to explore under our own steam and discover the fascinating houses, museums and culture of a formative period of American history.

Sadly, our American cousins did not always demonstrate the same appreciation. One such example was the small town of Saint Francesville, Louisiana. The first stop on the hop on service was the retail outlet on the edge of town, where the majority of passengers alighted. The rationale given by one woman electing not to go further was that she had already visited downtown San Francisco and had no wish to go back!

The second bus was used for excursions slightly further afield. One such trip was to the Civil War battlefields at Vicksburg (or *Myburg* as Vic/Vinny naturally renamed it). Within the 1800-acre site we made a number of stops for the guide to provide us with a plethora of interesting facts. We finally arrived at the *pièce de résistance* – the highest fort (raised ground rather than a building) in the Confederate lines, providing sweeping views across the battlefields and the Mississippi. Instead of us alighting the bus, a fifth-rate actor dressed as a battle-worn Confederate soldier climbed aboard and subjected us to a fifteen-minute soliloquy on the deprivations of life during the war. The Americans lapped it up while we stared out of the window and gritted our teeth. Then, to our amazement – and I have to say considerable disappointment – the bus departed. No exploration, no history, no photo opportunity!

Having arrived in New Orleans on the steamer, we were taken to our hotel via a three-hour bus tour of the city, with cemeteries featuring prominently, only to discover that our accommodation was a ten-minute walk from the dock. The tour guide spent the whole time describing past events using the present and future tenses. By the end I was literally banging my head on the window in frustration (as, we subsequently discovered, were the other Brit couple). But at least we then had three days on our own to absorb the magnificent wonders of the Big Easy before returning home.

I conclude my tales from the Deep South, not by 'Walking in Memphis' or gliding through the bayou handling baby alligators passed around by the tour guides. Instead, I thought it might be interesting to describe our visit to the fully functioning Louisiana State Penitentiary, better known as Angola Prison. A bit of a busman's holiday, given my profession, but it really did put the icing on a very nutty cake.

Angola used to be one of the most dangerous penitentiaries in the country. But the current warden has turned it round, using a faith-based system, to such an extent that wardens elsewhere are treating it as a model – and tourism has become one of its new income streams. The assistant warden, who showed us around, made it clear that he did not expect inmates to embrace the faith as long as they complied with the principles. At the time of our visit in April 2019 there were sixty-eight men on death row but executions had been suspended due to an inability to source the necessary lethal drugs. We were shown the now-disused execution block with its electric chair. Needless to say, some of our American friends had their photos taken sitting in the chair, grinning inanely. Luckily for them our vehement opposition to capital punishment, and strong humanitarian beliefs, meant that there was no fear of us searching for the switch.

The assistant warden explained how, at one end of the scale, they had inmates sentenced to two years' imprisonment. However, if they did not comply with the rules, a simple word with the judge would result in their sentences being increased to ten years! At the other end of the spectrum were many lifers. I tried to engage the assistant warden in conversation about the operation of life sentences in the UK. But it was pretty pointless as the idea of parole was a complete anathema to him.

We were shown the farm amid thousands of acres of open arable land, providing the penitentiary with self-sufficiency. There were no concerns about escape attempts as the penitentiary is surrounded on three sides by mountains and alligator-filled swamps. We saw a video of the annual inmates' rodeo that attracts thousands of visitors. Inmates are actively encouraged to take part despite a complete lack of training or any form of health and safety protection. Those volunteering to take part seemed to regard recovery from a few broken bones as a welcome distraction from the normal drudgery of prison life.

The tour finished in the chapel with a demonstration by a group of lifers who train assistance dogs for service veterans with post-traumatic stress disorder (PTSD). As part of the training, the dog is taught thirty-two commands, including ten specific to the veteran with whom the dog has been matched. Vinny was keen to discuss these commands with one of the lifers whose dog was called Issy – the lifer appeared to enjoy the conversation!

So, another fascinating insight into the American way of life, this time one aspect of their criminal justice system.

Based on this admittedly brief experience, I think I will stick to what we have in the UK, warts and all!

Although I have focused here on the weird and wonderful ways of our American brethren, I have to say that overall, they provided us with far more in terms of hospitality, friendship and entertainment than anything else.

Immediately following our return from the USA, I suffered excruciating pain in my neck. It was so bad that I was unable to lie down and had to sleep in a seated position leaning against the headboard. Not surprisingly, periods of rest did not last long and I frequently found myself downstairs at 3 a.m. taking my mind off the pain by watching old episodes of *The Saint* or *Randall and Hopkirk Deceased*. The mock-fighting scenes were so faux that I could not help but laugh.

Consequently, I made an appointment at my local health centre. Without any examination I was sent away by the locum doctor with a prescription for codeine and advice to put heat on my neck. This now seems quite incredible considering that medics believe my neck fractured, due to the cancer infiltration, on our return flight from New Orleans. That dismissive attitude caused me to seek assistance from the private osteopath co-located within the health centre. For the next eleven months, until my diagnosis in March 2020, I received treatment from her on a weekly basis – including manipulation!

Amazingly, my neck did initially feel as though it had improved and, assisted by copious supplies of ibuprofen and paracetamol, I just got on with life. Looking back and, inspired by Tony Hawke's splendid book about his travels

Round Ireland with a Fridge, I am beginning to wonder whether I should have entitled this book *Global Travels with a Broken Neck*.

Briefly adopting that theme, I have created below a list of some of the interesting things that I did in the space of less than a year with a partial disconnect between my head and my spine! It is quite a list, even though I may say so myself.

a) Four weeks touring Japan during the Rugby World Cup, covering ten cities/tours, eight hotels, international and domestic flights (including transits in Hong Kong), bullet trains, coaches, metros, boats, three sell-out rugby matches, a typhoon, two earthquakes and walking an average of six to twelve kilometres a day

b) following the 2019 Cricket World Cup in packed stadia in Taunton, Bristol, Southampton and Edgbaston

c) Test matches at an equally busy Lord's

d) following Bath Rugby on numerous occasions in Bath, Claremont and Belfast, the latter trip including a walk along the Giant's Causeway

e) walking over half the length of the River Wey in sections

f) cottage/walking holiday on the Devon/Dorset border

g) long weekends in the southern Cotswolds and Exeter

h) walking through Westonbirt Arboretum

i) continuing as a defence lawyer in Hampshire, Berkshire and Surrey, but also taking in journeys to Sussex and South Devon

j) dancing in the aisles at an Eagles concert at Wembley, and the Tina Turner musical in London; also seeing Francis Rossi in Aldershot and Jonathan Pye in Guildford

k) Leah's graduation at the University of Reading and post-celebration lunch

l) a long walk to, through and from a Christmas *son et lumière* at Kew Gardens.

I admit that my list does not include an FA Cup Final appearance at Wembley. Nevertheless, I must be nudging ahead of the late and great Manchester City goalkeeper, Bert Trautmann (who broke his neck during the 1956 final but carried on playing), if only in terms of the volume and diversity of endeavour! But unlike Bert's autobiography, I hope this focused memoir falls firmly within the humour genre!

I will elucidate on some of these adventures in later chapters but for now I just want to enlarge upon our River Wey walks. These came about after we had completed our objective to walk the full length of the thirty-three-mile-long Basingstoke Canal from Mapledurwell in Hampshire to West Byfleet in Surrey. This we undertook between November 2018 and March 2019. We did so by walking sections of three or four miles, enjoying a pub lunch and then returning to our car, thereby effectively walking the full length of the canal both ways.

I have to say that, apart from the wonderful weather and scenery we enjoyed, it was a real eye-opener. I have lived and worked in the area for over thirty years and yet found myself walking beside roads through towns that I had driven along countless times without appreciating that the canal was so close. I felt rather embarrassed.

We walked behind the Military Police Station in Aldershot, where I have spent many an hour, and through Woking town centre, a stone's throw from the court and the police station, to name but a couple of examples. The view from the towpath gave such a totally different perspective, and informative boards along the way provided excellent insights into the workings and history of the canal.

Harvey, our West Highland Terrier (Westie), accompanied us throughout, often modelling his designer "Mud" collection boots. Those booties did not go down well with his stylist but he scrubbed up well afterwards. He also sported his neckerchief when we reached the end of the canal, where it joins the River Wey, and toasted our achievement with a glass of champagne.

The confluence of the canal and the river was made stunningly romantic by the proximity of an M25 overpass, the South Western Railway mainline and an electricity substation.

Canal and river walking became a bit of a minor obsession wherever we went. For example, when in Toulouse for a Bath Rugby fixture, we walked the three kilometres from the city centre to the ground along the *Canal du Midi*.

Closer to home we next decided to embark on walking the River Wey. Although the canal joins the river in the middle of its course, we started our river walk at its accessible source at Godalming Wharf, Surrey. This was in April 2019 after our return from the USA. I could not understand why I was finding it such a strain in comparison with the Basingstoke

Canal. Of course, we now know that I had a fractured neck and cancer raging in my bones!

We returned to the towpath in July 2019 as the lure of the river outweighed the discomfort caused by walking along the towpath. By February 2020 we had made it as far as Send, but I did find it hard going and the distances I was able to cover became ever shorter. Again, I was surprised by the course of the river and the familiar sights it took us through and to, including Guildford Crown Court from an entirely different angle! We also circumnavigated the grounds of the sixteenth-century Sutton Place, formerly the home of John Paul Getty Junior but now believed to be owned by a Russian oligarch as evidenced by some fierce-looking guards and their patrol dogs.

Since the easing of Covid restrictions, I have managed to complete the towpath walk along the River Wey to the point where it meets the River Thames at Weybridge. I never thought that I would be able to do this with brittle bones and wearing a neck brace. My ambition now is to pick up the Thames Path at Weybridge and make my way, in stages, to the Thames Barrier. It is amazing to think that, starting just two miles from our home in deepest north-east Hampshire, it is possible to walk alongside canals and rivers all the way to the Thames Barrier and beyond – an uninterrupted towpath stroll of around 75 miles.

The last time we had walked alongside the River Wey, prior to my diagnosis, was on 18 February 2020, by which time I was really beginning to struggle. I was still seeing the osteopath on a weekly basis but now decided to seek a second opinion. I therefore arranged a consultation at the Royal National Orthopaedic Hospital (RNOH) in Stanmore on a private basis.

You can imagine my shock when, on 11 March 2020, a consultant spinal surgeon explained that my problems were caused not by an orthopaedic issue but by metastatic breast cancer and a related fracture in my neck. He immediately referred me back to my GP. By 17 March 2020 I was in Basingstoke Hospital.

3

The Zoo

At 8.30 a.m. on 12 March 2020 my GP rang me to advise that she had referred me to the oncology department at Basingstoke Hospital following receipt of the RNOH diagnosis that morning. I was then due to have an outpatient's appointment on the afternoon of 17 March 2020, but on the morning of that day my consultant oncologist, Dr Marcus Remer (who, for reasons that I will explain later, I now call The Thin Controller) rang to inform me that he was admitting me to hospital forthwith on the basis of my blood tests. Vinny was already performing brilliantly following my diagnosis, doing everything for me, just like Tonto does for the Lone Ranger. I therefore decided to give myself the nickname of Chemo Zappy.

Vinny took me to the Acute Assessment Unit at Basingstoke Hospital, as directed, where I was immediately placed on a fast drip because the calcium levels in my blood were rocketing. I remained on that drip for twenty-four hours by which time the pain that I had been suffering from for months just disappeared. If only I had known earlier!

That afternoon I underwent an MRI scan and, by mid evening, a bed had been found. Vinny came up to the ward to see me settled in – but this was only six days before the country went into the first Covid-19 lockdown and the hospital was already preparing for a sharp increase in coronavirus cases. Vinny was advised that from 9 a.m. the next morning, 18 March 2020, no visits would be allowed.

The bed they found for me was on E4, an endocrinology ward. I was in a six-bed, all-female bay and my arrival promptly brought down the average age by twenty years! It seemed that the other patients were suffering from dementia in varying degrees. The woman opposite was shouting, "Nurse, my back is killing me. Open the window, I'm so hot!" The window was open and she had a noisy fan as well. The woman diagonally opposite me kept saying something that sounded like, "Hit me, Hit me!" and my immediate neighbour was mumbling, "Dear God, Dear Jesus . . ." The woman next to her would not get back into bed.

I wondered how much sleep I would get that night, but regarded it all as just part of life's rich tapestry.

My prediction about the possible lack of sleep was spot on. It was all quiet by midnight. A nurse came to see me to give me a further drip – which would run till 6 a.m. – and some paracetamol. I thought, *Great, now I can just drift away.* I thought too soon. At 12.10 a.m. a doctor arrived and woke up Mrs Back Hurts for tests. Not surprisingly it all kicked off again. Her complaints about her pains and wanting the window open began to stream once more. This, in turn, caused Mrs Hit Me to wake up. Mrs Bed Escapee and the sixth woman, who at this point I had yet to name, so simply became Mrs Six, were now both trying to get out of bed!

By 1 a.m. the redoubtable nurses had restored calm and I felt myself dozing off. Suddenly I was jolted from my sleep by a booming, good-humoured voice approaching Mrs Back Hurts' bed. "Good Morning, Mrs xxxx! I'm the medical registrar." He proceeded to ask her a number of questions in a cheerfully loud voice. As I reached for my phone to check the time, the medical registrar said to the nurse, "She's a bit drowsy."

Too ****ing right, I inwardly screamed. *We all are!* It was only 1.40 a.m.!

However, I did feel sorry for Mrs Back Hurts. She was clearly in a lot of pain. After a great many tests, and sterling efforts by the nurses to make her comfortable, she was finally shipped off to another ward.

Not surprisingly, all the activity had woken Mrs Hit Me. I started to feel sorry for her too as, in between plaintive cries of "Hit me," I heard, "Please don't hit me," so I began to wonder about her past experiences. (I did raise my concerns with a nurse later but obviously would not know whether any enquiries were made.)

By 4 a.m. calm finally descended and I dozed off thinking how fortunate I was compared with some of my fellow patients.

Later that day, through a little light cross-examination, I ascertained that Mrs Back Hurts was upgraded to F floor. I seemed to recall that the situation was much worse up there. Vinny, Leah and I, together with my sisters and their families, had the joy of a week of visiting in 2017 when my mother was first diagnosed with dementia. She was on F floor. Unfortunately, she was a participant rather than a spectator so we never got to hear what happened during the night (except when my mother had a nightmare about the hospital burning down – but could not distinguish between dream and reality when relaying the details to us).

Awake again by 6 a.m. that morning, 18 March 2020, the entertainment continued to keep me occupied. Mrs Bed Escapee told Mrs Hit Me to "Go **** off, you dirty old git," and also called her a dirty, grimy shitbag. Mrs Hit Me continued her fake plea for flagellation, Mrs Bed Escapee remained abusive while Mrs Six was singing 'Dormez-vous'!

After my drip was disconnected, I was able to take myself to the loo. As I passed the nurses' station, there was one healthcare assistant (HCA) on guard duty. She looked stunned to see me walking towards her and asked if I was all right. I said I was fine and just going to the loo. When I returned, the guard detail had increased to five or six and all were looking equally stunned.

I commented that it must be rare for them to see one of their patients walking unaided. Or perhaps they thought that I had been quietly building up strength in order to make a bid for freedom. It was at this point that I thought to myself, *Welcome to the zoo.*

It was not long before I was taken off for a CT scan and then, after much discussion, a physio arrived to fit me with a neck brace and told me that I would have to remain on my back until further notice. (In hindsight I think the reason why the nurses looked so stunned when I made the trip to the loo was because I should not have been walking around with a broken neck. Little did they know the extent of my globetrotting over the previous year in said condition!)

Having to lie flat on my back brought with it the dubious delight of having to use a bedpan, something that I had never experienced before. At my first attempt I had a minor incident – a slight overflow due to waiting for its removal – sorry if this sounds like TMI! I did apologise by saying that I had previously been given a bladder transplant and that the donor was a bedwetter . . . but I am not sure that my black sense of humour was fully appreciated in the circumstances.

Thereafter I had a very refreshing bed bath until it got to washing down below. The procedure involved pouring a lot of water between the legs. I thought the fictitious bladder donor had gone into overdrive.

On 19 March 2020, following the analysis of my earlier MRI and CT scans, I was told that the neurosurgeons at Southampton General Hospital, with whom Basingstoke had been in constant contact, had decided that they would not be operating on my broken neck so I could move straight to radiotherapy.

By this stage I have to say that I was bowled over by the number of tests I was being subjected to, and the speed and efficiency with which they were being conducted. These included the bedside visit of a doctor at 9 p.m. the previous night to do strength tests on my arms and legs, for which I got top marks!

The flow of information and decision-making were also extremely impressive. In addition to being informed of the decisions taken at the earliest opportunity, the basis on which each decision was made was openly shared with me, including the rationale for going down one particular route in preference to the potential alternatives.

The staff were just wonderful. From the daytime HCA who regarded me as part of their team, and her colleague who cleaned my glasses without me having to ask. To the nurses and doctors (except the one who tried to take blood from my arm – never let a doctor take blood!). To the registrars and consultants, particularly an endocrinologist who was added to the list of consultants who thought that I am some sort of loon (tales of Luscious Doris, Chemo Zappy and all that!). He was flabbergasted that it had taken sixteen years for me to pop up on the cancer radar again – usually it takes no more than ten years for metastatic cancer to emerge, so I learned.

My session of radiotherapy was booked for the following day, 20 March 2020, at Southampton General Hospital. I was therefore able to look forward to being let out on day release from the zoo early that morning!

For comfort reasons, I had the joy of being taken on a stretcher in hospital transport accompanied by a member of staff riding shotgun. I certainly know how to travel. I was told that the plan was for me to be back in Basingstoke by about 4 p.m. My immediate thought was to hope they built some leeway time on the tag so that I could resume my newly discovered pastime of ward-watching and analysis without too much interruption. Vinny had offered to occupy my bed, claim squatters' rights and take notes for me while I was in Southampton.

Meanwhile I learned that my new temporary home, E4, was actually a medical ward specialising in diabetes. This explained why the consultant was an endocrinologist and the staff kept checking that I was not diabetic and did not need my blood sugars taken.

As evening approached prior to my day release, things once again began to warm up. Mrs Hit Me had just woken up, which would, in no time, set off Mrs Bed Escapee. Mrs Dear God thought it was the previous day. But early promise of entertainment soon faded – Mrs Bed Escapee shouted at Mrs Hit Me, "Who's on the phone? Put the phone down!" when it was actually me talking to Vinny.

The nurse came to me with the drugs trolley saying she was the new drug dealer. I responded by saying that she had come to the right person because I was a criminal defence lawyer and could represent her. The nurse was not sure what to say but Mrs Dear God burst out laughing.

During the night Mrs Alcohol, Mrs Back Hurts' replacement, was distressed but very quickly calmed by the wonderful staff. The recently arrived replacement for Mrs Six, who I had not sussed out given her remote position in the ward, needed assistance. She sounded very elderly but entirely with it. However, that opinion was not to last long. I named her Mrs Corner Job and she was a snorer. The combination of her snores and the noise of Mrs Alcohol's nebuliser disturbed Mrs Bed Escapee enough for her to start singing happily in her sleep. At 1 a.m. Mrs Hit Me stirred with a chorus of "Hit me, hit me; thank you," to which Mrs Bed Escapee replied, "You're welcome," and Mrs Corner Job just muttered, "Oh ****!". Trepidation hung in the air. (*Who let her in?* I thought in a moment of mild exasperation!)

By 6 a.m. I realised that I had had some sleep but wondered why I had woken up. Oh yes. Mrs Corner Job had managed to get hold of her table and bang it loudly. She wanted the radio switched off. Except the radio was not on. The less-than-dulcet tones she could hear were those of Mrs Bed Escapee. Mrs Corner Job then went in for a spell of call-bell ringing. Every time she pressed her bell it generated a noise in my corner. I drifted to sleep wondering if the reminiscent two-tone sound was an indication of the early arrival of the Black Maria to take me to Southampton.

Morning then broke in all its glory. The light was shining through the frosted glass and the previous Christmas's holly branch, snowball and robin were still decorating the window. The nurses started their rounds, checking oxygen masks and changing pads, replacing wet sheets. Naturally they left me alone, still trying to figure out what an oncology patient was doing on their endocrinology ward!

I was looking forward to my day out – a change of scene and the welcome light relief of some palliative radiotherapy. I thought my new grey hoodie PJs would be the order of the day – suitable for day release, provided they could get the hood over my neck brace. I did, however, wonder if I would get back to find myself in the middle of a scene from *One Flew Over The Cuckoo's Nest* with a stray Native American trying to throw a sink unit through the wall!

I was collected by two ambulance men for my transfer to Southampton. An HCA from Basingstoke accompanied me and remained with me throughout the whole day. I was grateful for this because Vinny was not allowed to be there due to the Covid-19 situation, but at least I was able to stay in constant contact with him during the day. The ambulance men used a spinal board to transfer me from my bed to a stretcher, as I was still confined to back rest. It really was like a scene from *Casualty* – on my count, one, two, three, slide.

My first stop on arrival at Southampton General Hospital was the *Mould Shop*. Here they made the mask that would protect my head when they administered the radiotherapy on my neck. The *Mould Shop* should also be known as the *Heath Robinson Cupboard*, given what they do there. It was in the cupboard that I saw an inspirational oncologist who explained to me that the object of the radiotherapy treatment was to kill the cancer cells in my neck. However, they obviously could not undo the damage that had already occurred. The neurosurgeons could not operate because there was no good bone either side of the damaged area to attach anything to. Basically, my cervical spine was shot and unstable, meaning I would have to wear a neck brace permanently.

After he left me, I admit to shedding a few tears. I was alone and in shock and wanted Vinny to be there. Momentarily I looked inside the dark box containing glimpses of what could have happened to me as I went about living a near-normal life, unaware that I had cancer and an unprotected broken neck that was deteriorating. I was horrified by what I saw – so firmly shut the lid of the box and vowed that I would never peep inside again.

Consequently, I have not for one moment looked back or asked *What if?* or *Why me?* I judged that that approach would only cause angst, particularly as nothing can be done to turn back the clock and change what has happened. I determined there and then that the only way forward was to be positive and adapt to a new way of living.

My moment of disconsolation did not last long. The oncologist had been so good in counselling me to think of the neck brace as a new integral part of my skeleton; it's just external rather than internal. He said that he had a cohort of women bedecked in neck braces under his care, who live their lives to the full. I somehow did not think, however, that his outside pursuits were on the same page as mine – when I mentioned live sport he laughed and said that he did not want to "yuk my yum"!

Having fully absorbed the essence of this pragmatic discussion, I had a further CT scan with mask on before being taken to the radiotherapy area. This was so far removed from the *Mould Shop* as to be unbelievable. It was a state-of-the-art area with six machines on the go all day. The mask was reapplied, pinning me flat to the machine so that I could not move. Time was then spent positioning me correctly before I was zapped either side of the neck for no more than a couple of minutes. A whole day spent prepping me for a few minutes of treatment – what service!

A radiotherapy department is essentially an outpatient one – and a potentially sombre one at that – so it must be unusual to have an inpatient there. They kept me and my HCA escort in an open area within the office space so that I was not mixing with any outpatients or the great unsanitised (due to the Covid-19 pandemic).

At one point I was laughing with my escort. A radiologist asked if it was me laughing. I immediately apologised but was told to carry on as it was lovely. The staff bought me bananas and orange juice out of their own money to keep me going.

It was a knackering day, not helped by transport issues for the return to Basingstoke from Southampton. The ambulance collecting me was severely delayed and, even as the ambulance men were wheeling me out, their control tried to re-route them. Having found myself, during lockdown, getting into TV programmes such as *Inside the Ambulance*, I now fully understand the pressures that they are under. Fortunately, a successful extension to the tag time meant avoiding the possibility of early evening unpleasantries fired by fellow patients on my return to the ward.

One of the side effects I was warned about from the radiotherapy treatment would be a sharp increase in pain for twenty-four to forty-eight hours. A forty-five-minute journey on my back on a stretcher in an ambulance ensured that such pain kicked in. On returning to the zoo, I successfully ran the gauntlet between Mrs Bed Escapee and Mrs Corner Job, despite Mrs Hit Me being in fine voice with a low accompaniment from Mrs Dear God. Even the ambulance crew were somewhat taken aback by Mrs Hit Me's Ian Dury impersonation and started to search for their rhythm sticks!

Having checked that there were, indeed, no Native Americans attempting to throw sink units through the wall by my bed I decided that discretion would be the better part of valour by gratefully accepting a *soupçon* of liquid morphine sufficient for pain relief but insufficient to constitute a chemical cosh. The dosage was perfect. It doused the pain but not my awareness, as I was later to discover when the sudden re-emergence of loud banging meant that Mrs Corner Job's table was back within her reach! Once the offending item of furniture was eventually removed from her grasp, and I lay back in a moment of rare relaxation, I found myself smiling when the brief silence was broken by Nurse Ana's open-mic question. Directed principally at Mrs Bed Escapee, Mrs Corner Job and Mrs Dear God, she asked which one had opened their bowels.

Suffice to reflect that the radiotherapy went according to plan and represented another step on my odyssey. Matron, in all her specialness, granted Vinny the rare privilege of a visit during the following morning, 21 March 2020. Like gold dust, and I am not going to divulge how many precious loo rolls and bottles of sanitiser I had to source on the Covid-19 black market in recompense.

The visit to Southampton was not a day to be frightened

of. Everything was so well explained and I did not experience any pain until my return journey to Basingstoke as I was forewarned. The oncologist told me that as soon as I was back at Basingstoke, I could sit up in bed – and that proved to be a huge plus. Another small step in the right direction. I could now prepare for the next steps and, metaphorically at least, walk tall (at five foot three, I am vertically challenged!). I reminded myself of my favourite motto: *Illegitimi non carborundum* – Don't let the bastards grind you down!

The morning of the 21 March 2020 saw Mrs Hit Me in full throttle for a couple of hours, but with Mrs Bed Escapee trying to drown her out with her own rendition of 'Deck the Halls'! I couldn't quite grasp the significance of this particular carol almost three months after Christmas!

I was distracted from such entertainment by Vinny's arrival, a truly wonderful boost; it was fantastic to be able to see him in the flesh. This may have only been my fifth day in hospital but so much had already happened. It was a non-contact visit but at least we were not peering at each other through a Perspex screen. He decided to join my soap opera in the form of Mr Suited and Booted. He developed the theory that, if he visited dressed in a lounge suit rather than a shell suit, or other similar apparel favoured by the likes of those who shop (or used to shop) in Asda, Farnborough, he would be better able to keep a safe distance from those still out on the streets living in Covid-19 denial, as well as the hoard of Coronavirus testees queuing up outside the hospital.

He also decided to wear his genuine US Detention and Deportation baseball cap, awarded by US colleagues when he was a director at the UK Immigration Service (now the UK Border Force), in the hope that it might give him a vague air of authority. The thinking was that his appearance would so discombobulate my fellow detainees that the ensuing silence would create an ambience more conducive to a quality visit!

Unfortunately, his carefully formulated theory backfired badly when he was frequently mistaken for a hospital consultant on entering the hospital grounds. He had to quickly design a name badge to wear round his neck on which he had inscribed MR SUITED AND BOOTED (EXTREMELY MAD AND VERY BAD). Moreover, the baseball cap had no impact whatsoever; indeed, it appeared to excite some of my fellow detainees into thinking that they were about to be deported to a better place. The visit of an apparent US immigration official also seemed to have brought back unwelcome memories for Mrs Hit Me!

Vinny's visit was followed by a most important event – the Celebration of the Presentation of the Self-control Panel for the Management of Mattress Position. I thought this worthy of suitable preparation so decided to wear my in-vogue purple and white striped gown with V-neck and capped sleeves. This was bulked out at the bottom by plenty of white cotton petticoats. Arm jewellery was very important. For my left arm I chose a very funky designed bracelet with two wavy tubes (cannula), and on my right a trio of flat coloured bangles, red (penicillin allergy), white (ID) and yellow (lymphoedema alert). Very fetching.

So, there we were. Staff Nurse Giulia was at my side, self-control panel in one hand, pain relief in the other and the ceremony passed without incident . . . well nearly. Unfortunately, the sudden unexpected release of four days' lack of bowel movement, probably assisted by the last wafer-thin cheese cracker consumed beforehand, almost earned me the *soubriquet* of Mrs Creosote!

Another event that afternoon was the flying visit of Doctor Roller Skates, winging in on his wheels. I am sure they must have written on my notes the following advice – *Just rock up, say hello, she will grin at you like a Cheshire Cat, hand-lob her a piece of* info – I should like to emphasise that they have never lobbed me any info with the pin still in! – *and then let her process it.* It was great because each bit of info provided to me helped form another piece of the jigsaw explaining my stay there.

Having checked I understood why I was there, he then explained why I was on an endocrinology ward. All inpatients have to be under the care of a medical consultant. Because I was an emergency admission I had to be placed where there was an available bed, in this instance on an endocrinology ward. Hence me being here under the care of a consultant endocrinologist.

That night I was fortunate enough to manage a few hours' sleep before being serenaded with '*Eine kleine Nachtmusik*' from Mrs Hit Me. But I did not mind being woken – it gave me the opportunity to reflect on the day's events, including Vinny's visit.

Overnight the wonderful Sister Ana was on duty (she of open-mic questions about bowel movements!). On arrival at the bay, she simply called out to me "Hello, Issy. Are you OK?" The following morning she just called out to me about taking my drugs. It was so good to be involved in a two-way discussion rather than being told what to do.

It was strange to be still in hospital on 22 March 2020 –

Mother's Day. Obviously, there were no visits due to Covid-19 and it was a quietish day for the campers, including Mrs Hit me and Mrs Bed Escape. While, strangely, I missed the shouts of "Dirty shitbag!" and renditions of 'Deck the Halls', it did mean that the wonderful staff were able to get on with their invaluable work without too many unwelcome distractions. I hoped that there might be some discharges in order that I could have some more characters to observe. Dr Roller Skates did his usual weekend flying visit, making sure I was all right, and that my steroid drug treatment had been halved, before skating off in a flash.

The Monday following Mother's Day, 23 March 2020, began with Mrs Hit Me warming up her vocal chords for another bout of fun and laughter. I was slumbering in relative peace on my bed, watching yet another episode of *Midsomer Murders* while the HCAs busily attended to various ablutions. I told myself that I really must get used to the idea that, in my new world, an HCA is a healthcare assistant and not a higher court advocate!

I had a visit from yet another inspirational oncologist. She explained that she was going to send me to radiology for a liver biopsy. This wasn't because they were concerned about my liver *per se*, but because it is the best organ to get tissue from in order to trace the path of the C blighter – where it has come from and where it is going – so that they can best plan my individual course of treatment going forward.

The consultant who conducted the biopsy was, needless to say, excellent. He decided to take two samples of tissue as I had done so well and he did not want me to come back. He paid me a huge compliment by saying that he did not think I looked nearly sixty and asked me what creams I used! He said, in the nicest possible way, that he never wanted to see me again.

When the porter arrived to whisk me off to radiology for the biopsy, all had been relatively quiet. On my return some while later all hell had broken loose. The Native American really was now trying to break out of the ward and Nurse Ratchet, having clearly given up any hope of wresting back control, was following suit. The ambient noise from Mrs Alcohol's nebuliser was not assisting. Mrs Corner Job was in the zone and must have transgressed while I was away because she appeared to have forfeited the afternoon promise of early parole. Mrs Hit Me was in the finest fettle yet, while Mrs Dear God was filing her nails! Given how the evening would pan out she really should have taken her opportunity at that moment to make a run for it.

As for Mrs Bed Escapee, she sweetly observed, as I was wheeled back past her into the bay, how nice it was that the empty bed space was being filled. I pointed out to her that I had been there all week but that nugget of intelligence was too much for her to process as she made yet another grab for her Zimmer frame.

Mrs Hit Me was in a fresh frame of mind. Instead of just lying there saying, "Hit me!", she was eyeballing Mrs Bed Escapee diagonally across the room and actively – and successfully – goading her into a reaction that included comments such as, "Shut up, I've got family too!" (?) and "I know you're not the full ticket but you should be ashamed of yourself."

Four hours later Mrs Hit Me was still going strong, having ground Mrs Bed Escapee down to limited shouts of "Shut up". Mrs Dear God briefly offered hope of a welcome change with a tune but sadly it was not to be.

By 10.30 p.m. calm was beginning to descend. Unfortunately, because I had had a local anaesthetic for my biopsy, I was on four-hour observations. Staff Nurse Giulia arrived with a machine to fix up to my feet – it was to help circulation as I had been in bed for a few days. Once it was attached, I looked as if I had just walked out of a Martian sweet shop – long green jelly tubes wrapped round my ankles and flying saucer wafers exploding alternately under the soles of my feet every ten seconds, to be continued throughout the night. I had heard this alien sound on previous occasions coming from Mrs Alcohol's bed space. Now I had one of those machines too. Not only did it work wonders for my circulation but also for wind, so by 2.30 a.m. I really had become a fully paid-up member of the zoo!

I must again express my eternal gratitude and admiration for our front-line workers at the NHS. What would normally take weeks, if not months, in terms of tests and treatments had been whisked through in a matter of days. I could not fault their attitude, determination, bedside manner and outright professionalism. These comments are not just restricted to Basingstoke, Southampton and Sarum Road, Winchester (where the oncology department later relocated because of Covid-19) but to Stanmore (Royal National Orthopaedic Hospital) where I sought that second, private opinion that led to my diagnosis. The oncologist who sent me for the liver biopsy said that seeking a second opinion had been absolutely the best thing I could have done when it became clear that the pain in my neck and shoulder would not go away. It was at Stanmore that I saw Mr Michael Mokawem, consultant spinal surgeon. We talked about Springbok rugby (although too close to England's defeat by South Africa in the 2019 World Cup Final for comfort!) as well as my condition, and it had been to Mr Mokawem that fell the difficult task of giving me the cancer diagnosis on 11 March 2020. But he did it with great empathy and professionalism, and followed up with truly caring and motivational calls about my condition and progress.

On 24 March 2020 I was informed that I was ready to be discharged. Strangely I felt a little tinge of regret as I prepared to leave my maniacal cocoon that was E4 ward to return to the wider infested world of Covid-19. I started to prepare myself for the journey home and to embark on the next stage of my odyssey (subject, of course, to the magical mystery tours to which hospital transport were already committed!). Physio came to see me and satisfied themselves that I would be able to get in and out of bed and walk up and down stairs without assistance. But my release had to be put on hold at the last minute because of issues relating to the need for my neck brace to be changed on a regular basis by someone suitably trained in the art once I had been discharged. Something of an anticlimax and disappointment!

That afternoon was very quiet. Mrs Corner Job had gone home, Mrs Alcohol had been shipped out to another ward and Mrs Hit Me was due to go as well. The reason for the sudden exodus was the decision to transform the whole of E floor into overflow wards for Covid-19, the country having gone into full lockdown the day before. The trouble was that, with it being so quiet, I could now hear Mrs Side Bay from beyond E4 shouting her head off in dismay as though she was in labour. It reminded me that I had heard this sound on previous nights, but had been confused as I knew that the maternity ward was in a completely different building. (The reason I knew this was because the last and only previous time that I had been an inpatient in Basingstoke Hospital was twenty-three years earlier for the birth of Leah.) I was just beginning to wonder what the night might have in store for me when the matron from The Firs, the specialist orthopaedic unit, arrived with a porter to transfer me there.

It was very strange being wheeled through a hospital that had largely been cleared in preparation for the anticipated Covid-19 influx. The empty corridors had a decidedly *Marie Celeste* feeling about them. I reflected that E4 had been in a very sad state of affairs when I left. Mrs Hit Me, Mrs Dear God and Mrs Bed Escapee were all flaked out on their beds, still waiting to be moved. Whatever happened to them I shall never know.

On arrival at The Firs, I found it to be peaceful and roomy in comparison. However, I pretty quickly realised that I had been hoodwinked. It was really a type of Darby and Joan facility. I anticipated that the activities manager would bound into the room at any moment, in the guise of Coco the Clown, and expect me to sit in my high-back chair, grin inanely and clap along to the music.

Once formal introductions had been completed, I soon understood that my new bay inmates, Didi and Gogo, were only capable of making disconnected statements about their personal situations and medical history. There was no chance of them being able to weave such statements into a meaningful conversation. As if to prove the point, when advised that I was only going to be there for one night, Gogo responded by saying that she would behave as though I did not exist. That suited me as I was able to withdraw from any frustrated attempt at polite conversation and leave them both to wait for the alternative person destined to fill my bed space who was never going to arrive!

All was not lost, though. Poor Didi seemed distressed at around 5 a.m. I called out to her and she explained that she could not find her bell. So I was able to summon help for her using my own bell – my good community deed for the day (or night)! That being said, I was mightily glad that this was not a foretaste of the type of *community* that awaited me on my release.

Despite the issues my fellow patients may have had, I cannot fault the overnight treatment that I received. On my final morning a delightful older night-shift HCA brought hot tea and said she would shortly start bossing everyone around. I asked if that included me and she said, "No, you can sort yourself out!"

Then Vinny arrived, not just to transport me home, but also to receive tuition on how to change my neck brace, there being no community physio available to do so on a regular basis at home (presumably because of Covid-19 and lockdown). The neck brace consists of two parts, back and front, held in place by strong Velcro straps. It has to be changed at least once a week in order that the foam linings to the hard plastic can be washed. I have to lie very still on my back while Vinny undoes the Velcro, removes the two parts to the brace, replaces them with another brace and resets the Velcro straps. I can basically carry on with my mobility as before – I just have this new bit of external skeleton to assist me. I have been repeatedly assured that, provided the collar is on, I will not have any difficulties. It must never come off except when Vinny the Technician performs the weekly swap. Fortunately he passed the training tests at Basingstoke Hospital, both practical and theory, with flying colours!

Once back home Vinny, having never cooked during the twenty years of our marriage, decided it was time to launch his new chef's chain, *Vogg Victuals*. It is because of his newly acquired cooking skills that he earned the *soubriquet* Vinny the Pinny (and it is through this that the nickname of Vinny emerged).

Over the following months he transformed himself into a variety of additional characters depending on the nature of the task in hand. These included Vinny the Hort, the jobbing gardener; Vinny the Chauffeur, who ferried me to my numerous medical appointments; and Vinny the Coiffeur, who attacked my hair with scissors before it retreated in a mix of terror and chemo-induced hibernation. It was not long before the name Vinny had ousted that of Vic in a bloodless coup in the minds of our circle of family and friends.

Vinny's culinary productions on my first day at home were a smoked haddock chowder for lunch and a fish pie for supper, both based on recipes from the *Royal Marsden Cancer Cookery Book*. They were really delicious, and I had seconds at both sittings! But in order to cook, one needs ingredients, so I would like to pay special thanks to our wonderful neighbour, Tamsin, who shopped for us in the early days of lockdown before I was able to get myself registered as a vulnerable person and arrange priority slots for home grocery deliveries. When Tamsin delivered those first few bags of shopping, it gave me the opportunity to observe social distancing for the first time. She and Vinny seemed to be dancing some strange slow fandango on the courtyard while I lobbed unhelpful comments through the open breakfast-room door!

That evening I went to bed at about 9 p.m. I was exhausted, not because of feeling ill, but simply lack of sleep. I woke up after five good hours of sleep, curled up in my normal sleeping pattern, laughing at myself. What had I been thinking about when I went to bed? I had laid down carefully on my back, in a pristine straight position like a tin soldier. Did I expect some ethereal observation machine to come alongside and latch on, pumping me full of oxygen and life? Of course not. I returned to sleep, waking up later again smiling at my gift of life and laughter.

Mind you, I do not think Vinny thought it much of a laughing matter. He was convinced that my last night in the Darby and Joan Firs Club had been a ruse. In reality I had been roaming the wards on E floor like something out of *The Bodysnatchers*, looking for the zoo patients so that I could bring them home to keep me company. As I had drifted off to sleep, he was hanging plaits of garlic and ceremonial rhythm sticks over the bedroom door.

It was such a pleasure to be back home with Vinny. Naturally it was very disappointing that Leah could not be there as well due to Covid-19 and my new vulnerability. But she and our Westie, Harvey, had relocated to the house of our friends, Judy and Nigel, five miles away in Alton. They had so generously offered to absorb them into their protective social bubble pending a return to near normality. Little did we know at the time just how long that would turn out to be.

My immediate focus, meanwhile, was on getting my strength back, adapting to my changed circumstances and embarking on an effective treatment plan, whatever form that might take.

4
The Shunting Shed

Having been discharged from hospital on the morning of 25 March 2020, I now had to get used to the sudden and permanent change in my life. Initially I was very weak and struggled to get up and down the stairs. Vinny would walk in front or behind me to ensure that I did not fall. Obviously, I had to get used to wearing the neck brace but have to say that Vinny very quickly became a dab hand at changing that for me. Pretty quickly, whenever I thought about my neck brace, all I could see in my mind's eye was my neck being supported by a pile of gold rings as worn by Queen Nefertiti. Therefore, naturally, I named my first collar, Nefie.

But my alternate needed a name too. Vinny, in his own inimitably wicked style, suggested that its Formula-1 type streamlining made it synonymous with waking up next to Lewis Hamilton – or so he imagined! I could not have a neck brace called Lewis so I asked for suggestions on my Odyssey Facebook page. A theme quickly developed relating to giraffes and, in particular, to the tribal women who wear neck rings similar to Nefertiti. I therefore decided to name my second brace, Stretch. I even persuaded Vinny to put a Tippex blob on the back of Nefie so that I would always know which one I was wearing. Sad, I know, but I thought that if I had gone to the trouble of naming them, I should at least be able to tell them apart.

I have to say that giving my second brace the giraffe-related name of Stretch was much to Vinny's consternation, given the traumatic memories it evoked of his namesake, Victor the giraffe. In 1977, Victor attracted international media attention after collapsing at Marwell Zoo, Hampshire. His legs splayed out and, despite a number of ingenuous attempts, nothing could be done to lift him to his feet. Keepers presumed that he had been entertaining his partner, Dribbles. Sadly, Victor did not survive but the happy ending is that later that summer, Dribbles did give birth. Although Vinny said lessons have been learned from this unfortunate incident involving his namesake, he still has the occasional PTSD flashback! But he soon came to terms with the giraffe-themed name of my second neck brace!

The next phase of my treatment was due to be discussed with my oncologist, Dr Marcus Remer (The Thin Controller), at an outpatients appointment at Basingstoke Hospital on 3 April 2020. A couple of days beforehand it was necessary for me to attend my local health centre for blood samples to be taken. This was a fascinating but successful visit. It was run like a military operation, no doubt fine-tuned in the light of experience since lockdown began just a couple of weeks beforehand. Dr Diligent had directed that I be at the front door at 10.40 a.m. precisely. I was assured that there was no appointment before or after me so I would not come into contact with any other patients.

On arrival I could see that in the entrance between the inner and outer doors there was a table containing gloves, masks and hand gel. I rang the bell and Philly the Phlebotomist appeared to let me in. Having both gelled and masked-up appropriately, we retired to her office. Philly did the necessary and within minutes we were back at the front door.

At this point there was a slight, unexpected hitch. Vinny the Vigilant was out of the car on observations when he spotted an odd-looking couple who, having misread the daily operations order directing no attendance at the surgery without prior appointment, were camped outside the front door in masks and gloves blocking my exit. Vinny subsequently told me he was about to shout at them to Foxtrot Oscar, but before he potentially let the side down with such oafish behaviour, Philly opened the door and, in no uncertain terms, told them to move and let me out. They scuttled off and kept their distance. I am sure that as I exited the building for the car, I saw Private Walker of *Dad's Army* fame, eyeing up the black-market, high-value contents of the gel and glove table in true spiv-like manner.

With blood tests taken and the results safely conveyed to my oncologist, Vinny and I happily set off for my outpatient appointment at Basingstoke Hospital on 3 April 2020. Vinny had created a sign explaining that he was TAKING CANCER PATIENT TO MEDICAL APPOINTMENT to hold up to the driver's window should we be stopped by an eager traffic officer demanding to know what we were doing out and about during lockdown. But we barely saw another vehicle on the roads. It felt like we had strayed on to a set of *War of the Worlds* where suddenly a Covid-19-infected Martian might crash-land in front of us.

Once at the hospital we faced something of a logistical challenge. Vinny dropped me at the main door before going to find a parking space. The first test on his return was to avoid a group of smokers hanging around the front entrance and failing to observe social distancing. Creeping along the walls to the lifts, we operated buttons with our elbows and made sure we had the lift to ourselves before embarking.

Once in the oncology department we met The Thin Controller for the first time, but without actually seeing his face as he was socially distanced on the other side of the room and masked-up alongside his similarly attired assistant, Chief Engineer Empathy.

It was at this consultation that he explained the seriousness of my situation. Not only were there spots of cancer on my lungs and liver but it was widespread in my bones. It was in my spine, femur and hips, was extensive in my pelvis and had spread to my breastbone. In addition to my neck fracture there were further fractures to my ribs. The bone damage was considerable with some actually destroyed.

The Thin Controller provided me with the outcome of the various scans and tests that had been undertaken in a clear and factual manner. We held our spectacles in front of our faces to see the horror show that was unfolding on his computer screen on the other side of the room. The Thin Controller asked whether I wanted to hear the prognosis. I did, of course, to which the reply was, "Six months – perhaps longer with treatment."

I must have completely blocked this death sentence from my mind as I searched for something more positive to cling to and The Thin Controller began to talk about treatment options. We could start, he explained, with gentler hormonal treatment or a course of chemotherapy. For the latter he had in mind a drug called Paclitaxel, which would be administered once a week for eighteen weeks. I have since discovered that this drug is more usually used in a palliative setting for those who have already had a course of chemo. There was no way I wanted to shilly-shally around with softer options. "Bring on the chemo," I told him. "I have no intention of shuffling off this mortal coil anytime soon."

As we were about to leave there was a lock-in as a corona convoy rumbled down the F-floor corridor outside. All the staff were suitably attired in suits and masks such that I felt that we had stepped into a remake of *E.T. the Extra-Terrestrial*.

Once we were released, I commented to Vinny that I thought the consultation had gone well and had provided us with a very positive base from which to work. Although he kindly agreed with me at the time, he later admitted that he thought he had suddenly entered some parallel universe that left him wondering whether we had both been at the same meeting!

That afternoon The Thin Controller rang me to say that he had reviewed the proposed course of treatment and discussed it with senior colleagues at Southampton General Hospital. He was now proposing a more intensive course of chemo using two drugs, usually used in a curative setting, one of which was Epirubicin or EP for short. EP is the same as Doxorubicin, the Red Devil, the strongest and nastiest chemo drug then on the market. It has to be administered extremely carefully as any spillage will cause untold damage to surrounding tissue, either externally to the skin or internally if the vein breaks. The revised regime was to be administered every three weeks over an eighteen-week period. Fortunately, no such spillage occurred at any time during my six cycles.

I only told Leah about the original prognosis after I had completed cycle five of the six-phase round. She responded in true Leah style – "**** me, Mother. You'd have only just scraped sixty. Now you can really enjoy your birthday!"

(Which is exactly what I did when 16 August 2020 arrived, but more of that later).

The following day, 4 April 2020, the oncology department of Basingstoke Hospital moved, along with that at Winchester Hospital, to a combined department at the private BMI Sarum Road Hospital, Winchester, in order to better protect cancer patients from the threat of Covid-19. As a result, the newly named Rainbow Unit at Sarum Road soon became my second home.

We live not far from the Watercress Line, a restored heritage railway line where, on high days and holidays, Thomas the Tank Engine and friends can be seen trundling up and down. The Fat Controller strikes an imposing presence at one of the few stations along the route. In a moment of whimsical reflection, when visiting the Sarum Road hospital for the first time, I suddenly transported my new situation into the world created by the Reverend W. Awdry and began to see everything in a Thomas the Tank Engine setting. Basingstoke Hospital became the mainland and Sarum Road, aka ChemoWorks (South) Ltd, transformed itself into the new shunting shed on the Island of Sodor. Each time on arrival at Sarum Road, outpatients are required to go through Check Point Chemo, a form of triage screening for Covid-19, along with various other tests. I immediately thought of the cancer patients as engines, the nurses as engineers and the sisters as chief engineers. Not surprisingly my oncologist, Dr Marcus Remer, became The Thin Controller. The Shunting Shed took wings (in a matter of speaking).

My first visit to the Shunting Shed was on 7 April 2020 for my initial cycle of chemotherapy treatment. After successfully negotiating Check Point Chemo, I was met by duty Engineer Compassion, who took me through to the engine room. This spaciously housed ten tenders/tanks all having their systems cleaned up. I was seen by The Thin Controller, who fully explained the clean-up process to me before it was administered by Engineer Compassion.

The whole atmosphere was very positive. Mrs Wig, a second timer, and Mrs Mallard were discussing alternative covers for their chimney stacks. At that point I felt sure that when I attended for my second cycle, I would be joining in the various conversations like an old hand. I managed to avoid guffawing with laughter when Mrs Fairy Queen, positioned next to me, responded to preparations being made by one of the engineers for her cancer injection by saying "Cancer? I didn't know I had cancer!"

My visit to Sarum Road provided another brilliant example of the professionalism and dedication of the NHS. This was the first working day of the newly located department and it was short-staffed because of Covid-19. One of the nurses attending me had come out of retirement. Yet they carried on regardless and I could not admire them more or thank them enough.

My next trip, to the Odiham Health Centre for blood tests on the 24 April 2020, generated a good deal of excitement, but only because it was the first time that we had been out of the house in the seventeen days since my first cycle of chemo. It said something about lockdown that we started to look forward to my medical appointments.

Once on the open road, the first thing that struck me in the great outdoors was the glorious yellow colour of the rapeseed in the fields around us. Next, I was taken aback by the amazingly long queue for the farmers' market in Odiham High Street. Actually, there were only about a dozen people in the queue but, because of social distancing (a concept that I was still unfamiliar with), it seemed to stretch forever.

Again, the health centre was highly organised. This time I had to use the rear entrance from where I was collected by the masked and gowned Philly the Phlebotomist. She remarked on how cheerful I was.

All processes were completed in about five minutes. I saw no one else in or near the surgery except for a lone soul in the adjoining public car park, using the bottle bank. I could understand the collection of full bottles being classified as an essential activity during lockdown, but not disposing of the empties!

Three days later I was back out again, this time to head off to the Shunting Shed for the insertion of a PICC (peripherally inserted central catheter) line. This is a line inserted into a vein in the upper arm with the end of it finishing just above the heart. Apart from the sting of the local anaesthetic I felt nothing. It meant blood could be taken from it, and the chemo drugs injected through it, so there would be no more needles in my arm or cannulas in the back of my hand. Joy!

The following day I returned for cycle two of chemo. The engines present were a little more morose than previously and I did not think any of them were in the mood for me to start a knees-up. Mr Born-in-48 opposite me seemed more interested in the hot drink and biscuits, and devoured them as if he had just been rewarded for donating blood. Maybe that was what he thought he had done! My engineer sat with me for an hour using huge plastic syringes to insert the two drugs intravenously through my PICC line. Some of my dependent clients back in the criminal justice world would have been in seventh heaven if they had been able to use syringes of that size! All went well and I left with such a concoction of follow-up drugs that I could start my own pharmacy.

During cycle two my Denosumab injection was delayed for a couple of days. This is a subcutaneous injection, designed to improve bone density, that I receive every twenty-eight days. In essence, the Denosumab works by transferring calcium out of my bloodstream and directing it into my bones. Alongside the Denosumab I take daily calcium supplements to replace the calcium in the bloodstream that the Denosumab extracts. The delay to my latest injection was explained in a call I had received from The Thin Controller's sidekick, Dr Stinchcombe. (Her ancestor Linfred – also an ancestor of Harry Potter – invented the potion Skele-Gro!) My blood calcium level was evidently too low to have the injection. ("Regrowing bones is a nasty business," as the nurse said to Harry Potter!) So Dr Stinchcombe upped my munching of calcium tablets to increase the levels in my blood and enable me to have the jab alongside cycle three of chemo. I quite like the calcium tablets – they are like extra-large Dextrosol sweets!

The trip to the Shunting Shed on 19 May 2020 for the third cycle was very amenable, particularly on the back of my conversation with The Thin Controller the day before when he had explained to me that my treatment was going as well as could be expected. One liver test was back to normal. The other, which is more specific to bone cancer and where normal is 120 or below, had come down from 900 to 300. My kidney test was fine – I had been dehydrated, but no longer. My calcium level was down slightly, as explained above, and I was slightly anaemic, but that was a normal side effect of the treatment. My platelets were normal as was my protein. Most amazing of all was my tumour marker, which is one of the tools used to gauge how the treatment is going. Normal is 30 or below. Mine had been at 1066 before treatment started! Now it was down to 160.

The Thin Controller was also pleased that I remained pain-free, despite my neck and rib fractures, and was therefore able to get by without pain killers. (In the months prior to my diagnosis I had been chomping my way through them on a regular basis.) Consequently, he was able to give me the green light to go ahead with cycle three the following day, along with the Denosumab injection. The Thin Controller also decided that my next CT scan would be after cycle four, whereas normally it would be after cycle three.

Once inside the Shunting Shed for cycle three, I noticed that there were two newbie engines in attendance. Mr Ambidextrous was in the chair next to me, to my right. He was asked whether he was left or right-handed and replied by saying he was both but mainly used his right. His engineer put all the procedures in his left hand/arm. She then needed him to fill in a form, at which point he said he wrote with his left hand so she had to assist him. He was clearly very anxious and, as an old-timer, I wanted to give him a bit of reassurance. But the combination of the chair positions, my neck brace and being hooked up to a saline drip in my left arm through the PICC line ahead of chemo being administered, made that impossible.

The other newbie, Mrs Bravado, was diagonally across the room from me. She appeared to be putting on a brave face but was also anxious, particularly about the self-administered injection that we had to give ourselves on the day after chemo to prevent infection, an anxiety with which I could fully relate. I really disliked having to do this but took the view that as there were plenty of children with conditions such as diabetes who regularly have to inject themselves, why should I not be able to do so? Again, as an old-timer, I wanted to give her some reassurance but it would have meant shouting across the room, which I did not think was appropriate (and not my style anyway)!

I did see The Thin Controller briefly while parked in the Shed. I said, in response to his question, that I was feeling chilled, particularly after the promising telephone conversation we had had the previous day. This provoked half a bashful smile in his eyes – he was, as always, wearing a mask.

I was back at the Shunting Shed on 19 June 2020 for cycle four. Once taken through to the full inspection area, I was assigned my engineer for the procedure. There was no sign of The Thin Controller but I knew he was always there in the background. Mrs Chatter was next to me. I did not get an opportunity to talk to her directly because we had the same engineer who was alternating between us. She was explaining to the engineer how her son's post-uni travel plans to go to New Zealand had been thrown into a spin back in November 2019 because of her diagnosis. Initially I thought she had been in chemo for a long time. But it then dawned on me that either she had had pre-surgery chemo, followed by surgery and was now in post-surgery chemo, or that she had been unlucky with time slippage in her cycles. But either way, like me, she was very cheerful.

Mrs Shy sat next to her. A couple of times she made eye contact with me as if she wanted to speak, to which I smiled in response, but the face masks made it very difficult to read facial expressions! Plus, as I have mentioned before, the chairs are socially distanced. It took my mind back to my inpatient time in the E4 Zoo at Basingstoke Hospital. My main fear fortunately never came to pass – namely that I would wake up in the middle of the night to find Mrs Bed Escapee next to my bed peering at me, reminiscent of Edward Rochester's wife escaping from her tower and staring at Jane Eyre!

In the opposite corner was Mr Double Check. He had obviously had some issue with his medication and was verifying dosages. It is funny how all of us, me included, will quite casually discuss our respective medication and procedures in a manner enabling all other engines in the inspection area to tune in should they so wish!

To my surprise a packed lunch was brought round at 11.15 a.m. It included an egg sandwich (à *la* Japanese 7-Eleven stores, referred to in a later chapter), crisps and chocolate sponge cake – not particularly healthy I feared! I left the Shunting Shed clutching my untouched lunch bag together with a much larger bag of medication referred to by two different engineers as my goodie or my party bag.

Vinny was delighted to see me carrying lunch that had been prepared by someone other than himself. He suggested that we might celebrate this – and our short window of freedom – by having a picnic in a lay-by on the A33 *en route* home. However, we decided to put all romantic thoughts to one side given the obvious need to stick rigidly to our social isolation responsibilities. Instead, I simply climbed back into the pneumatic tube that transported me home without passing Go or collecting £200.

On 15 June 2020 I had to attend Basingstoke Hospital for a CT scan. This was the first time that I had been there since The Thin Controller had donned his black cap with his six-month prognosis on 3 April 2020. I was met in the CT department by radiology assistant Vlad (real name). Well, of course, I immediately dubbed him Vlad the Impaler. He explained the procedure, which included inserting a cannula into the back of my hand to inject an iodine contrast. Given the moniker that I had just attached to him, I was so pleased to learn that he would not be the one assigned to sticking sharp objects into my hand!

A charming radiographer came along to do the procedure. Vlad had forewarned that when the iodine contrast is injected, it causes a warm sensation. As it happened, I suddenly found myself humming the tune to Ed Sheeran's 'Bloodstream' and thinking again of Vlad; I wonder why! I was in and out within the hour. Vinny the Chauffeur waited in the car park but came up to meet me at the main entrance. Jobsworth, the security guard, told me to put my mask in the bin. I refused to comply with his direction, explaining that I needed to continue wearing it due to my vulnerability. What a rebel I am!

In between my three-weekly visits for the administration of chemo, I also had to attend the Shunting Shed on a weekly basis for my PICC line to be cleaned and dressed, as well as to have my blood tests and Denosumab injections. On one such visit during cycle four I arrived just as numerous other engines from Sodor converged. Mrs Nuisance demanded her husband park right outside Check Point Chemo, thereby blocking it for all others. This act of selfishness resulted in Mrs Anxious, who was just taking her seat, being separated from her sister, Mrs Stress, who was raising the temperature on the other side of the vehicle by seeking to enter the Shed as well.

I calmly stood back, socially distanced, explaining to Mrs Stress that she would not be allowed in. Mrs Nuisance, who had by now taken her seat, decided to chime in loudly and reiterate to Mrs Stress that entry would not be permitted.

I was invited to take my seat leaving Mrs Stress pacing outside. Her behaviour was clearly causing distress to Mrs Anxious, whose respirations were causing concern to her engineer. I sat, observing, with an enigmatic smile on my face while Mrs Nuisance was triaged. Once completed, instead of fully leaving the ante-shed, she once again blocked the entrance by chatting to Mrs Stress. She even ignored the engineer who deliberately walked between them with hands outstretched indicating that they should be standing further apart.

Mrs Glum had to slip round the side of them and, in doing so, managed to queue-jump. One of the engineers apologised, saying she would be with me shortly. I told her not to worry – I was chilled.

Well, I certainly was not wrong there – they thought I had chuffed in on a cloud because my steam (blood) pressure was so ridiculously cool. I was cleared to go.

My visit to the Shunting Shed on 30 June 2020 for cycle five followed on from the now-traditional conversation with The Thin Controller the previous day, when he had confirmed that the cycle could go ahead. He was also able to discuss with me the upshot from my CT scan on 15 June 2020. The cancer in my bones, which was extensive, had improved everywhere – pelvis, lumbar, spine and neck. He was still surprised that I was not in any pain and that I had not taken any form of pain relief since leaving hospital in March 2020. There was still a long way to go but my bones had filled in a bit, where much had been destroyed, and the damage, which was considerable, had reduced. It was very pleasing to hear this, particularly as I recalled my thoughts when I saw my first CT scan in March 2020. Then I had asked myself where my neck was – instead of white bones there had been a grey amorphous mass.

There was also considerable improvement in the liver. The two cancerous spots had reduced in size and my liver blood tests had improved significantly, returning to normal. The two tiny nodules on my lungs were unchanged, which led The Thin Controller to believe they were non-cancerous. He was unconcerned about them. My tumour marker was now down to 97 against a norm of 30 and starting point of 1066. As for my white cell count, he stated that this has always been within the normal range.

The Thin Controller confirmed that this was all very positive and that I was "in the best place possible". Consequently, he was now able to formulate a post-chemo plan – not something that could have been considered previously.

So, once at the Shunting Shed on 30 June 2020, I successfully negotiated Check Point Chemo. Inside the main doors, the chairs in the waiting room were suitably spaced as always. Fellow patients sat quietly minding their own business and waiting to be called . . . except for Mrs 4x4. I have so named her because of the amazing frequency with which Vinny and I find 4x4s parked close to us, invading the motor equivalent of personal space, when we return to sparsely populated car parks. Mrs 4x4 certainly had no spatial awareness, irrespective of social distancing. She walked past my chair so closely that she almost touched me and I involuntarily shrank from her. She did not just do this once but three times in close succession. Fortunately, I was collected before I could say anything I might later regret.

Chief Engineer Charming administered cycle five. We had a good laugh while she did so, particularly as she referred to the EP drug as my injection of rosé wine. How apt for a wine lover – I would always now think of that connection! I also admitted to her for the first time that I called the unit the Shunting Shed and that my oncologist was The Thin Controller. She found that hugely funny.

Another engineer asked how my Facebook blog was going. There was also another pleasant newbie who was most taken with the headwear covering my chemo-induced baldness, so I had to give her the website details.

When I first started the course of chemo, I was provided with the emergency number for the acute oncology ward and advised of a number of symptoms to look out for, such as a high temperature, which might indicate infection. With a compromised immune system, the concern was always that an infection might cause neutropenic sepsis, which can be fatal. Such a call would result in telephone triage and, if necessary, an ambulance would be sent to collect me for admission and immediate intravenous antibiotic treatment. I mention this just to give an indication of the serious issues that the acute team might have to deal with on a routine basis.

Fortunately, I did not have to call them for this reason. But I did have to for reasons of my own making. At the Shunting Shed, prior to the administration of the chemo drugs, I took anti-sickness medication. For the first four cycles this caused the uncomfortable side effect of constipation over the first weekend; I will spare you any more details. Consequently, for cycle five, The Thin Controller prescribed different anti-sickness medication that I was then required to take at home on the following two mornings.

On the first morning I mixed up my new anti-sickness pills with my steroids. As a result, I inadvertently took two anti-sickness tablets instead of one. Whoopsee! As each tablet was 80mg, and the maximum daily allowed dose was 125mg, I had OD'd by 35mg. I immediately realised my error and called the Shunting Shed, who provided me with the mobile number for the duty engineer. That happened to be Chief Engineer Charming who had administered the chemo on the previous day. Fortunately, she was not unduly concerned, given the nature of the medication, but she indicated that she would check out the position with the pharmacy and the acute team.

She called back a few hours later, not only having spoken with the aforementioned services, but also The Thin Controller himself. She repeated the general lack of worry at my error but provided me with a list of potential after-effects to watch out for. Thankfully none emerged and, more to the point, I did not suffer the particular side effect that I had done in earlier cycles. I found it amazing that a little tweaking of medication can make such a difference.

I also received calls on the next two mornings directly from the acute team to check on my welfare. Such service for what, after all, was my own mistake. I had caused them unnecessary work by my own careless error but the follow-up, all charm and equanimity, once again demonstrated the care and professionalism of the NHS, for which I will be eternally grateful.

Vinny the Dispenser decided he needed to keep a watchful eye over my medication to prevent further lapses.

Our next trip to the Shunting Shed was on 17 July 2020 for PICC-line dressing and blood tests. We took the scenic route so that Vinny the Chauffeur could use his newly acquired app at the Shell garage to pay at the pump, thereby socially distanced and safe. We really had stepped into the twenty-first century with our use of apps, Zoom and other remote technology.

It was obvious, on arrival at the Shunting Shed, that fake news had emerged about future Russian intentions to hack into hospital treatment records. Check Point Chemo was extremely busy with engines lining up in a socially distanced queue. Poor Mr Dodder was struggling to recall his date of birth, while Mrs Glamorous had obviously confused the words *cannula* and *catwalk*, given her totally inappropriate mode of dress. Mrs Vacant arrived on NHS hospital transport for day admission. Because of her frailty she was immediately given a seat in triage by the driver. The looks of consternation on the faces of those waiting in line clearly indicated that this altruistic act on the part of the driver had engendered thoughts of queue-jumping. Instant assurances to the contrary had to be given.

Once inside, Engineer Efficient advised me that I would need to shield at home for four more weeks after cycle six, which would take me nicely up to my big Six-0 on 16 August 2020. He also explained that they like to keep the PICC line in for a few days after administration of the final cycle of chemo drugs, just in case of complications. He told me about Mrs Obstinate who insisted on her PICC line being removed immediately after the provision of the drugs. Two days later she was in the emergency unit with sepsis – no PICC line available for speedy intravenous antibiotic treatment. I wisely concluded that I would not be putting myself in that position.

My sixth and final cycle of chemo was administered on 21 July 2020. On arrival at the Shunting Shed, Check Point Chemo was empty and I floated in with a steam pressure of 125/85. Vinny maintained I had ice in my system.

On entering the main building, I was once again recognised without giving my name, despite still looking like an urban guerrilla, given my penchant for wearing scarves round my neck brace, along with head gear and face mask. It was a bit like going to the local, but being greeted with "A hundred and thirty ml of Epirubicin, Issy?" instead of "A large glass of Pinot, Issy?"!

I was treated by an engineer that I had not met before. She was a couple of years older than me and shared my black sense of humour, so we laughed our way through the proceedings. Another engineer called over to enquire how my Facebook blog was going. Having then explained the blog to my treating engineer, she suggested that I name the ward manager, who I had also not met before – The Fat Controller. The next thing I know a rather portly sister came over to me with the opening comment, "You can call me what you like!" I was mildly embarrassed as it had not been my idea to call her The Fat Controller, but a delightful conversation ensued during which she complimented me on my attitude and progress.

As I got up to leave, my engineer announced to the room that it was my last chemo session. I received a round of applause and much well-wishing – it was really quite moving.

A couple of days later I returned for the removal of my PICC line. I left Vinny the Chauffeur in the car park and walked the short distance to the main entrance, clutching my locked box containing all the used needles from those self-injections that I had not enjoyed. This had to be returned for safe disposal and as I gripped it tightly, it did occur to me that I never thought for one moment that I would ever enter the murky world of sharps and scripts inhabited by many of my clients.

Check Point Chemo was empty apart from two engineers, one of whom was Engineer Chatty, who advised me that he would be performing the PICC-line removal procedure. He departed inside to prepare while I underwent my triage tests. All were very good: temperature 36.7, sats 98, pulse 90 and BP 124/69 – despite feeling excited about the purpose of my visit!

Chatty was quick to collect me from reception. As I was saying goodbye to my PICC line, I thought I would take a photo of the visible part of it for posterity. I did, however, decline his offer to video the process.

Chatty did go on to explain that he had removed the line from a bowel-cancer-suffering former colleague, who had videoed it and uploaded it to Facebook. This then appeared on Chatty's page, which in turn was seen by another colleague, an infectious diseases nurse. Her comment was, "That's an interesting way to remove a PICC line." He had cleaned the area *before* removing the line, rather than *after*. He was quick to assure me that he was now fully up to date with procedures, and I have to say that he was very efficient and professional. He whipped the whole line out without me feeling a thing.

Because I had not observed the insertion process, I was really surprised to see that the line was about eighteen inches long. He then warned me that removal of the remaining tag might hurt a little because he had to cut out the two small barbs that held everything securely in place. It did pinch and sting a little, which made me wince, but nothing more than that and it was all over in seconds. I was back in the car within fifteen minutes, depriving poor Vinny of partaking of his flask of hot tea.

During each of the six cycles of chemo I did suffer certain side effects, but took the view that they were a necessary evil. After a couple of cycles, I soon worked out the course the side effects would take. Each cycle lasted three weeks, with the first day always being on a Tuesday when the chemo drugs were administered. For the next couple of days I would feel hyperactive, requiring Vinny to don his tin hat. This would be followed by the constipation and fatigue kicking in over the weekend. Thereafter I would bounce back and feel generally fine until starting another cycle.

However, there were two cycles when additional side effects emerged that were positively weird. Over the first weekend of the first cycle I felt completely fatigued, coupled with a peculiar but strong feeling of *déjà vu*. It related to everything – moving around the house, watching television, reading the online newspaper and so on. I felt like a visually impaired woman in a darkened room, searching for a black cat that wasn't there! Fortunately, in subsequent cycles, the strong sense of *déjà vu* did not reappear.

But then, in cycle six, it was the Cornish pixies! This cycle undoubtedly fuelled my most extreme bout of hyperactivity. I did recognise, of course, that the effect of the drugs might have been exacerbated by the thought, bordering on euphoria, that all six stages had been completed on time. I was awake throughout the first couple of nights following chemo – my mental filing cabinet looked like it had been burgled, drawers pulled open, papers everywhere! Then on the third night, while still hot-wired but beginning to calm down, I spotted some Cornish pixies hiding in the corner of my mental study, waiting for my metaphorical back to turn so they could tidy up their mess. Happily, the following night, the emboldened Cornish pixies came out of their corner and tidied up my mental filing cabinet. I just hoped that they put all the papers back in the right order so that I could find them easily when needed next.

The following day fatigue set in but I found that useful because it allowed time for the Cornish pixies to put their poles bearing knotted handkerchiefs on to their shoulders and march out of my mental study. The cabinet drawers were shut, table tidy and door firmly locked. I have not had any problem with Cornish pixies before or since – apart from a few days later when, as a result of a bizarre dream, I woke up feeling as if a couple of rogue pixies, accompanied by some troublesome elves, had broken back into my filing cabinet and located the stash of Tramadol that I had refused to take when in hospital in 2004 for my mastectomy because it made the walls move!

But it did remind me of one of my drug-dependent clients whom I represented many moons ago. When asked by the magistrates for an account as to why he had failed to attend court on a previous occasion, he explained that a giant green frog had been blocking his bedroom door and he had been unable to get out. It was accepted as a reasonable excuse!

The last day of my eighteen-week course of chemotherapy treatment was on 10 August 2020. On that day I had an excellent visit to an auxiliary Shunting Shed in Old Basing, otherwise known as The Hampshire Clinic, where I had been treated for breast cancer in 2004 and was now attending for a CT scan.

It was quite busy with a constant stream of engines chuffing through the MRI/CT scan area. But no one wanted to make eye contact with me, and Mrs Uncomfortable clearly felt decidedly awkward sitting opposite me with my bald head and neck brace exposed in all their glory. It was a very hot day and far too sticky for Vinny the Chauffeur to wait for me in the car. He therefore grabbed Harvey's dog blanket and sat in the shade in the hospital grounds. The scan went according to plan and I was soon back out again.

When I started my first cycle I was stepping into the unknown and the completion date seemed so far into the future. Yet, looking back, it had actually passed quite quickly.

I'd had no idea how I was going to cope with the chemotherapy treatment. I had set myself my own little target at the outset, which was to complete all six cycles back-to-back without any slippage. I have to admit that, in reality, I thought it would be surprising if I met my target. But I had and I felt pretty chuffed about it.

Now I could have a few weeks' break from treatment until my next meeting with The Thin Controller on 14 September 2020. The purpose of that consultation was to review progress and discuss the next phase of the treatment plan, a phase which could not have been contemplated back on 3 April 2020 when he had given me that initial dark prognosis. But I was now ready and willing to embark on the next stage of treatment. Bring it on!

However, I first needed to reflect on who I am and how I got to this point.

5

Who Am I?

I am the youngest of three sisters, a child of the Sixties. During the Second World War my father, Jack Dailley, was an officer in the 8th Gurkha Rifles, a unit of the British Army later subsumed into the Indian Army following India's independence. He spent much of the war on the North-West Frontier, now the Khyber Pakhtunkhwa region of Pakistan on the border with Afghanistan.

For a short time, he was a Japanese prisoner of war (POW) but, exactly how or where he was captured, I am not entirely sure. Like many of his generation and experience, he spoke very little about it.

One thing I did learn from him was that, as the senior British officer in the POW camp, he was singled out for attention. He had a V-shaped scar above the bridge of his nose, which I know came from a Japanese rifle butt. He must have taken some punishment on behalf of his Gurkhas because, when the guards scattered on liberation, the men went after them and, much to his hidden horror, brought him back the commandant's head!

My father contracted polio while serving in the army, and although eventually invalided out, he did not return home after the war until 1948. His last job before leaving the army had been an administrative one related to the Nuremburg trials. He made no secret of the fact that, had he not been invalided out, he would have remained in the Army. Had he done so, the three of us might have been Pad Brats, the nickname given to children of service personnel stationed at various British Army garrisons in the UK or abroad.

But his wartime experiences could not suppress his mischievous sense of humour, which has to be seen in the light of a post-war Britain, before political correctness and social media domination. As children (in a time long before Amazon) we remember he and a close friend arranging for unwanted parcels to be delivered to each other's houses. The *gifts* became more outlandish as they tried to outdo each other. Eventually their wives had to put a stop to it when toilets and piles of manure turned up unexpectedly on respective doorsteps.

He and another friend amused themselves on their commuter journeys by loudly discussing false information to see how long it would be before someone stepped in and corrected them. One of their favourites was to discuss how to get to Ewell West in Surrey. They wrongly pronounced it "eewell" instead of "uwell". It worked every time with some pompous commuter correcting their pronunciation!

He was a great raconteur and joke teller. One of his favourites went as follows.

When Noel Coward died and went to heaven, he was extremely excited to meet up with the Bard – Shakespeare. The conversation went like this:

Coward: "Mr Shakespeare, Mr Shakespeare. I'm so delighted to make your acquaintance. But tell me, darling, what is the secret of your success? How is it that, so many hundred years after your death, your work is still studied and revered the world over?"

Shakespeare: "Ah, Mr Coward. I can help you there. It's all in the rhyming couplet. See that man standing over there? Describe him using a couplet."

Coward: (rubbing his chin pensively for a few minutes) "Under yonder chestnut tree
A bandy-legged man I see."

Shakespeare: (shaking his head in dismay) "No, no, no. That won't do at all. This is how the couplet should read –

*Forsooth, what style of man is this
Who wears his balls in parentheses?"*

My father loved rugby and cricket (I wonder where I get it from!) although he never recovered from taking my mother to a Calcutta Cup match between England and Scotland at Twickenham. She fired off a whole host of questions in a loud voice, including one about the identity of the odd man wearing black with the whistle!

He was a great family man and very mild-mannered, but mention of the Japanese would cause a change. I recall once, when I was a teenager, the shock on my mother's face as my father unexpectedly drove down the drive in a new car. It was a Datsun, precursor to a Nissan. On being questioned as to why he had bought a Japanese car, he snarled – completely out of character – something unrepeatable about forcing the Japanese to work hard!

I hate to think what he might have said about our tour of Japan for the Rugby World Cup in the autumn of 2019, particularly our very positive feedback on the friendliness and hospitality of our Japanese hosts!

In much later life he developed Parkinson's Disease, which was then aggravated by the latent effects of the polio. He died in 1995, eighteen months after being diagnosed with prostate cancer. I still miss him, and his wonderful sense of fun.

While watching the commemorations for the seventy-fifth anniversary of VJ Day in 2020 I raised a glass to him. I was, however, somewhat dismayed by the misleading comparisons made at the time of the commemorations, especially in some parts of the media, between the risks and quality of life encountered during the Covid-19 lockdown and the situation in Britain during the Second World War. While both events are clearly tragic, to put it mildly, there are some unique differences between the challenges faced, deprivations suffered and overall loss of life during 1939 to 1945, and those associated with the Covid-19 lockdown, that do not bear direct comparison.

Having signed up in 1940, aged seventeen, my father's first civilian job after leaving the Army post-war was with the Hong Kong and Shanghai Banking Corporation (affectionately known then as the Honkers and Shankers and the forerunner to what is now HSBC). He did not remain in banking long, spending most of his career working in freight-forwarding, ending up as general manager of a company based at Heathrow Airport.

My father possessed the Midas touch when it came to raffles and tombolas. He rarely came away empty-handed. I recall one cold, snowy New Year's Eve when we had been to a smart function at Wellington College in Crowthorne. He won a rather magnificent bottle of gin in the raffle and, on leaving at the end of the evening, he slipped in the icy conditions. Rather than concerns being expressed for his welfare, he was met with a chorus of "Mind the gin!" This he managed to do with a great deal of unorthodox dexterity.

He applied his inherent luck, along with a good dose of logic, when playing fruit machines in the pub. Having watched others feeding the machine he would suddenly stand up and take his turn. Invariably the machine would pay out, he would collect his winnings and sit down. I never saw him put any winnings back into the machine.

Many years later I tried to emulate him while in Las Vegas. I was marginally successful, but could not live up to his standards, and I have not touched a fruit machine since.

My mother, Ann Dailley (nee Milburn) was at Sherborne Girls boarding school during the Second World War and subsequently went on to gain a degree in art from Leicester School of Art, later part of the university. Post-graduation she obtained a job with Harrods, her desire being to use her artistic talents to become a window dresser and move into fashion. Sadly, and as a reflection of the times, that avenue was only open to male employees.

From there she moved to the same bank as my father, where they met. Once they became engaged, one of them had to leave – because married couples were not allowed to work there together. As was the norm in those not-so-far-off days, it was the woman who had to resign.

They married in 1953 and settled in Little Bookham near Dorking, Surrey, before moving to Wokingham, Berkshire, where I spent the majority of my formative years.

Having left banking in order to marry, my mother initially worked in a local corner shop. Once I began schooling at the age of five, she spent the next twenty plus years running a nursery school, but combined that with bringing up me and my two older sisters, Philippa and Kate.

Following retirement, my parents moved to a small Hampshire hamlet, where they developed a vibrant social life. This continued for my mother after my father's death in 1995 until she developed dementia and moved into a care home in 2017.

My parents placed great emphasis on ensuring that their three daughters took education seriously and worked hard to reach their full potential. We attended the local primary school, where the headmaster was a progressive type, preferring a freer approach to education consistent with Britain in the Sixties. He allowed and encouraged individuality – for instance he did not punish my middle sister, Kate, for leading a full-blown march with placards around the playground, demonstrating against the poor quality of school meals. Kate won the day.

Unfortunately, my first experience of his approach landed me in significant difficulty. The teacher in reception class took an unfair dislike to me. The reason was quite simple. She was old school and did not appreciate the headmaster's methodology. He had introduced the Initial Teaching Alphabet (ITA) to assist learning to read. To clarify, this relied on a phonetic alphabet with about ten vowels, including diphthongs, which supposedly made it easier to learn to read. Because I could already read before going to school, I had no problem in following the ITA system. As a result, the head was constantly pulling me out of class to read to visiting parents to demonstrate the strengths of his preferred reading system.

It was not my fault that the head was deceiving them by deploying a pupil who could already read, but the reception teacher took it out on me.

The instruction we were given in class when answering a question was to raise our hand and wait to be asked – definitely *not* to shout out the answer. I vividly recall an occasion when the boy next to me (I even recall his name!) got overexcited and, as he put his hand up, shouted out the answer. His excitement spread to me and I did the same. But I was the one, not him, who was sent out of class for disobedience. I can still see myself in the mini ablutions, sobbing my heart out, not because I had been disciplined but because of the unfairness of the situation. Undoubtedly, in the longer term, this played to my advantage by sparking in me a strong sense of justice. It is no coincidence that I went on to become a solicitor specialising in criminal defence work!

On stepping up from infants to junior school, every morning would involve English and maths lessons with time allocated for sport in the afternoon. The rest of each day was spent individually completing work assignments set on a Monday for the rest of the week. I would always crack on and finish my assignments by Tuesday so that I could bum around during the time set aside for such work from Wednesday to Friday.

Strangely – or not – that approach to getting on with essential tasks in order to maximise the amount of time more directly within my control, has never left me!

As part of the headmaster's progressive approach, in 1968 he took a group of seven- and eight-year-olds to Normandy for four nights to see the Bayeux Tapestry. A memorable trip. We stayed in a typically small, family-run French *pension*. I had to share a double bed with a friend. The pillow was an old-fashioned bolster roll. All very peculiar to me at the time.

We were served with *moules marinière*. The majority of the

group turned up their noses, but little was wasted because I hoovered up their portions as best I could. So began my love affair with *moules* (sadly no more due to a seafood allergy developed in later life).

The actual viewing of, and affection for, the tapestry has stayed with me to this day.

The following year the headmaster organised another trip, this time to the Netherlands. We had a wonderfully rough crossing on the hovercraft from Ramsgate to Calais with the majority of other passengers looking decidedly green. We visited the tulip fields in Keukenhof, the potteries in Delft and the Euromast in Rotterdam; again an unforgettable trip. I always thought the headmaster was a wimp for being too scared to come up the Euromast with us. In adult life I began to have some sympathy for this as I suffered under the mistaken belief that I had developed an illogical fear of heights.

In using the word *illogical* I do not mean in relation to the fear itself, as many people are similarly affected, but more to the way it manifests itself. I have been up many tall buildings such as the Space Tower in Seattle, the Willis Tower in Chicago, the Empire State Building and, sad to reflect, the Twin Towers in New York, the Eiffel Tower in Paris and the Tokyo Skytree without any anxiety or discomfort. This, I believed, is because I have felt safe and secure within such structures. When I think back to the Rotterdam Euromast, I remember feeling safe for the same reasons. Take away that sense of safety and security provided by the fabric of a building and my anxiety levels increase dramatically, often regardless of the height involved. For example, I had to descend the Leaning Tower of Pisa almost as soon as I had climbed to the top. I have stood on castle walls just six feet off the ground and felt decidedly wobbly. My challenge in walking round Dubrovnik's city walls was to ensure I kept my eyes shut without falling over the side, such was the feeling of dread. Yet, paradoxically, I felt safe on the Great Wall of China, but setting foot on any glass viewing platforms in buildings that I otherwise considered secure would represent a step too far!

Bridges can be tricky too. They have an element of safety because of the parapet but they are often very open. In August 2018 Vinny and I took a thoroughly enjoyable trip to Lisbon and Porto. While in Porto I forced myself to walk across the top level of the Luís 1 Bridge and sent pictures to Leah to prove I had done so. Her response – "Mum, you look terrified!", which, of course, I was.

Consequently, I have always qualified my fear of heights with that of a feeling of safety. While having to shield during the first Covid-19 lockdown in 2020, I researched my so-called qualification online. To my surprise I discovered that I do not have a fear of heights (*acrophobia*) but a fear of falling (*basophobia*). Apparently, it is a natural fear and is typical in most humans and animals in varying degrees of extremity. It encompasses the anxieties accompanying the sensation and the possibly dangerous effects of falling, as opposed to the heights themselves. That exactly sums up how I feel.

Subsequently, my research paid further dividends when a related question arose on the BBC TV quiz programme *Eggheads*, compered by Jeremy Vine. Not only was I able to shout out the correct answer, but I also learned that *basophobia* and *phonophobia* (fear of loud noises) are the only two congenital phobias. The rest are behaviourally acquired. So, at the age of fifty-nine, I discovered something about myself. They say every day is a school day.

From primary school I moved to the local grammar school. Once again, my sense of justice came to the fore, particularly on the occasions that I was form captain. One year our classroom was a terrapin hut on the edge of the playing fields. During break we accidentally sent a ball up on to the roof. We decided it needed to be retrieved so two girls scaled the side of the hut. On swinging out to give themselves final leverage to get on to the roof, they put their knees through the top window. We had all been involved in the prank. I therefore believed it unfair that only those two who had actually broken the window should be punished. Consequently, I took the punishment instead by refusing to name them.

Acting responsibly was not my only task as form captain. It also fell to me to lead the mischief-making. A fun and regular activity was during French lessons. The teacher was weak and ineffective. I would give the signal and the whole class would gradually shunt their desks forward so that we were all scrunched up behind the teacher. Then, on the second signal, we would all shunt backwards to be scrunched up at the back of the room. The teacher carried on regardless as if nothing had happened. During one of these sessions, a classmate threw her pencil case out of the window, then climbed out to retrieve it. On coming back in through the door, she said, "Sorry, Miss, I dropped my pencil case out of the window." The teacher never questioned her on how she had managed to exit the classroom in the first place without using the door.

By the time we got to the Sixth Form I was not the most popular of students with the staff. In place of a head girl, we had six school stewards voted for by the students. I was voted in, much to the chagrin of the staff – so much so that they wanted the vote reconsidered in Donald Trump-like fashion. They did not succeed in changing their own rules to achieve a more palatable result – because that would have been unjust!

My days at grammar school fuelled my desire to travel, built upon my primary school travel experiences. The years 1975 and 1976 saw me experience two German exchange trips, largely brought about by my home town of Wokingham being twinned with Nidda near Frankfurt.

In Nidda, I became friends with Harry the postman, and spent time racing around, helmetless, on the back of his motorbike. Fortunately, the one time he came off his bike was when I was not with him.

While there, the big German chart hit was Frank Zander's 'Der Ur-Ur-Enkel von Frankenstein'. Find it on YouTube. It's a classic!

My grammar school in Wokingham was called The Holt. A terrorism-related incident in Forbury Park, Reading, in June 2020 resulted in the tragic death of one of its teachers. I posted my condolences on the Holt School Facebook page. It is not something that I would normally do, but I felt compelled to on this occasion by the particularly distressing circumstances. I am, as always, hopeful that some good will emerge from tragic events such as this and it was moving to see just how united the school community, both past and present, became in its response.

On a personal level, I was delighted to have become reunited with my earliest and closest school friend, Jane, as a result of the Holt School Facebook exchanges.

Jane and I have known each other from the age of five through our primary and secondary years. Sadly, we lost contact once we left school – no mobiles or social media back then! She has been living in Canada since 2013 and now, thanks to twenty-first century technology, we have reconnected. Of course, the little grey cells started churning and took me back to the idyllic, innocent times we spent in the Sixties and Seventies.

My family lived in a house in Wokingham, called *Summerleys*, in the unadopted (by the highways authorities) Tintagel Road, off Kiln Ride, where Jane lived. We spent much time at weekends and holidays together. On reconnecting via Facebook, I immediately recalled an occasion when we had placed milk and bread out for the hedgehogs in Jane's garden. We disturbed one and it got up and ran away. I blurted out, "Oh, it's got legs!" Well, of course it had legs – I had just never seen one run like that. What did I think it had – wheels?

Talking of wheels, a friend's father assisted in taking us to and from Sunday school. He had a Volkswagen Beetle and would fly along our unmade road with far too many kids in the back, who were joyously screaming at being thrown around. Not sure *Elf and Safety* or safeguarding would have approved had they been in existence at the time!

In our own garden I remember playing croquet and – using buckets and sticks – setting up space hopper gymkhanas. Such innocence – no video games then. While playing, we would hear the Corona (not coronavirus) lorry driving round like an ice-cream van. Bottles of fizzy drinks were a treat. Given that my grandfather was a dentist, I was surprised my mother allowed it.

Also, while in the garden and beyond, I was able to play on my Raleigh Mark 1 Chopper bike that I won at the age of ten in my first and only national competition success. I had to design an advertisement and strapline for Kellogg's. (Other breakfast cereals are available.) A quick look on eBay suggests that the bike in good condition would sell today for £1,200!

The entrance to the garden was through a wooden five-bar gate. Every day the milkman would use our driveway to turn his milk float round. One day in 1966, he misjudged it and smashed into the gate, damaging it beyond repair. Naturally the dairy agreed to replace the gate . . . so my father chose the most expensive one that he could find on the market. In 1988 my parents sold *Summerleys* to developers who intended to demolish the bungalow and develop the site. As the gate would be surplus to requirements, I took it (much to the dismay of the developers, who had obviously spotted its craftmanship). In 2021, fifty-five years on, it still graces our driveway. How many people can claim that one of their physical reminders of a childhood home is a wooden gate!

Another great friend from school, who I also lost contact with, was Sheela. Out of the blue in September 2018 she found me through Facebook. Neither of us could work out how, as she did not know my married name. We subsequently spent time taking walks and having lunches together. The intervening forty years just fell away. Sadly, in February 2019, she was diagnosed with cancer and died in September the same year but, happily, we had that small amount of time back together.

While growing up we were also lucky enough to have a selection of pets. One I recall was a kitten rescued by my eldest sister, Philippa. We named her Cleethorpes, or Cleo for short. At the time we had two West Highland Terriers, Haggis and Oliver.

Haggis was a grand old dame, placid as anything. Oliver had been the runt of the litter, totally feisty. Once we had coaxed Cleo off the top of the curtains and she had become used to the dogs, a definite pecking order emerged: Haggis at the top, then Cleo, and Oliver very much at the bottom. Cleo used to box Oliver around the ears and he just accepted it. On the other hand, Cleo would jump out at Haggis from behind a bush but Haggis would continue plodding along, completely ignoring the fact that there was a cat hanging round her neck.

As young children we had a Beagle, Candy. She had been rescued by my parents from neighbours who had kept her in a kennel at the bottom of their garden and, because the husband used to wear a long overcoat, Candy hated men in overcoats. On one occasion we had a visit from an electricity meter man. He walked down the drive in his overcoat and Candy started circling him. My mother, who was only a few feet away, told him to stand still and she would take Candy away. What did he do? He kicked the dog! What did the dog do? She bit him! Thereafter we got a snotty letter from the electricity board about keeping our dog under control.

Growing up we also had two other cats, Lucy and Polly. Lucy decided to jump ship and went to live with an old lady down the road who kept putting food out for her. Polly lived to the ripe old age of nineteen before, with some sort of death wish, she ran behind the car just as my father was reversing it. He was mortified. Strangely, since leaving home, I have had an allergy to cat fur.

In the garden we had a very large ornamental fishpond, which, as well as containing ordinary goldfish, also had an impressive selection of koi carp. I am not convinced that my mother really appreciated the frequency with which my father would arrive home with a new fish. Sadly, one summer, a strange fungus more or less wiped out the whole stock. My eldest sister, Philippa, organised the fish graveyard and day after day, the three of us could be seen in a line, Philippa at the front and me at the back, traipsing across the garden to perform yet another fish funeral.

Another aspect of growing up were holidays. Despite my good fortune at having experienced school trips to France, the Netherlands and Germany, overseas travel was rare. Package holidays abroad were still a thing of the future and not a prerequisite for having a great summer break. We had some wonderful childhood holidays, particularly in Cornwall with family friends and their children, Sue and Neil. On one occasion Neil and I, then both aged five, thought it would be a great idea to take an early morning stroll along the beach. We were found a considerable time later, well on our way from Downderry to Seaton. Oh, the consternation we caused! But my father got his own back on me that evening by placing a very realistic-looking rubber snake in the bath.

Frequent visits to Mevagissey were always fun. Whenever my sister Kate stepped into the sunshine she would be dumped on by the seagulls, causing the rest of us much merriment. The connection with Kate and animal excrement was most intriguing. It seemed that whenever we drove past a field full of cows or sheep, one would be doing its business and, of course, Kate had to point it out.

Crackington Haven, near Tintagel, was another favourite. Vinny, Leah and I visited there in the Noughties during one of our cottage holidays. Standing admiring the view from the cliff top took me straight back to my childhood, which really surprised me. We would always leave home at around 5 a.m. as it would take us all day to get there. No A303 then. Heading down the A30 we would only be at Andover before asking, "Are we there yet?" Needless to say, we would get restless. My father frequently slammed on the anchors, saying that if we did not behave, we would turn round and go straight home.

Games of 'cricket' with pub signs kept us going for miles. This involved gaining 'runs' by counting the number of legs in an animal or person found on a pub sign. Such simplicity. No electronic or in-car games.

Once into my teens, holidays had a different look. There was the boating holiday on the Thames when we managed to split all the side fenders, run aground on a sandbank and nearly lose my mother in the weir while mooring up at a lock. Even now I can picture time standing still, with us all holding our breath, as she rocked back and forth on the groyne, trying to regain her balance.

In Lampeter, Ceredigion, the locals all switched to Welsh when they heard our voices and my father was horrified to discover the whole place was dry of alcohol on a Sunday.

The rented cottage in Portnacroish, near Fort William, was barely more than a crofter's hut, where we had to dry our wet clothes on an old-fashioned clothes dryer in front of the fire.

While exploring castles in Aberdeenshire I felt most grown up getting squiffy on vodka and lime at a local *ceilidh*.

One of my lifelong passions has been following sport. As I mentioned earlier, I can only presume that this love must have come from my father because I have to fess up to the fact that my spectator enthusiasm has never been matched by physical ability, which has at varying times been described as ineffectual, accident-prone and even downright laughable.

My first recollection of the accident angle was at primary school during rounders. There was never enough equipment so the rule was to hit the ball, drop the bat and run. The girl in front of me, in her excitement, overlooked this and reached third base with bat still in hand. Unfortunately, her slinging ability exceeded her batting. The returning bat cracked me across the bridge of the nose – I suffered nosebleeds well into adult life.

I wanted to play football but that opportunity did not extend to girls in the Sixties. Weirdly, our progressive headmaster encouraged us to play shinty, an aggressive but fun Scottish Highland game. Apart from that it was netball. I could never get the hand-to-eye coordination, unlike Leah who once, when playing for her school, Farnborough Hill, banged in thirty-three of the thirty-six goals they scored in one match. Awesome!

Swimming was a disaster. I did not learn until I was ten, by which time I was, of course, aware of the dangers of water. Lessons were rigid and formulaic, failing to take into account individual ability or lack thereof.

Having barely mastered the basics of swimming we moved on to diving. A racing dive led to a belly flop, then guess what – a nosebleed. The torture continued at grammar school where each week we had to march crocodile-style to the local outdoor lido. Grim. I suffered from athlete's foot and frequently had to stay out of the water. Amazingly, that affliction cleared up the day I left school!

Also at grammar school, we had the joys of cross-country running and athletics. During cross-country, in Jubilee Park opposite our school, I would hide in the bushes part way round and wait for the returning crowd on the circular run.

I did, however, find a bit of a niche in field sports – discus, javelin and shot-put, representing the school in the latter. But I was alive to the fact that I was probably the only one willing to do so, and participation was not aided by my sister Kate referring to me as Geoff Capes, a high-profile British shot-putter at the time!

My temporary refuge during cross-country runs – Jubilee Park – contained one of the sirens for the maximum-security Broadmoor Hospital. Every Monday morning at 10 a.m. the sirens were tested and sounded just like a wartime air-raid warning. The sirens would activate for two minutes, immediately followed by a two-minute all-clear siren. In the event of an actual escape the siren would sound and there would be an immediate roll call of the whole school. Following the roll call pupils would leave by prearranged means – either waiting for collection by parents or taking the bus to be met by a parent at their destination stop. To my recollection there were two or three escapes during my time at school. They created a certain amount of fear and I shall always remember the look of shock on teachers' faces when the siren sounded unexpectedly. On the last occasion a number of Sixth formers, who had bunked off early, were seen scrambling back into school in time to meet the roll call.

From grammar school I moved on to Kingston Polytechnic, now University, where, on the sporting front, I fared a little better, probably because I could choose a particular sport rather than be directed. By my own admission I was pretty good at squash. A friend at school and another at Kingston were county players, so I had some useful tuition. But then injury found me at Kingston Hospital with cortisone injections and physio for grazing on the back of the kneecap.

Laughably perhaps, given my lack of hand-to-eye coordination, along with my lack of height, I was in the Kingston Polytechnic Ladies' Basketball team. I was useful at dribbling. We used to practise against the men's teams from different faculties – I just went underneath rather than around them.

I also played mixed rugby. Only the girls could score tries, which kept us in the game. I always seemed to be the one to receive the ball on the restart and ended up at the bottom of the ruck. I wonder why that was!

Post higher education I turned my hand to mixed hockey. Ironic, really, as I hated it at school – having to run around on a cold February afternoon in a short-sleeved Aertex shirt and gym slip while the teacher stood in her tracksuit, scarf, hat and gloves. As an adult, the enjoyment came from always having fixtures on a Sunday morning, thereby ensuring we could be in the pub for lunch. I also played darts for the local pub but, by mentioning that, I do not want to start a debate about whether darts is a sport or not.

During my academic years I was always keen to have part-time employment. My first job in 1971, at the age of eleven, was delivering papers every morning for the local corner shop, earning the princely sum of £1 per week. I even carried on with that job despite their German Shepherd dog taking a chunk out of my calf.

Aged fourteen I moved on to a Saturday job in a shoe shop. Between the ages of sixteen and eighteen I worked on Saturdays and in school holidays in a department store in Bracknell, firstly in the customer and staff restaurants and then in the soft furnishing department. There was nothing you could not tell me (please excuse the double negative) about working out the drop of patterns on material required to make curtains. So much easier these days (or at least it was) to have John Lewis make them for you.

As soon as I turned eighteen, I obtained a job in a local hostelry and, throughout my time at Kingston and later when I moved to the Guildford College of Law, I worked there during my holidays and at weekends when I could. I always had first dibs on choice of shifts until one holiday when the landlord directed which shifts I should work. I was a bit miffed but did not argue about it. A couple of weeks later he explained to me that one of the bar staff had their fingers in the till. Knowing it was not me, he was using me as a control. Having identified the tea leaf, normal service was resumed and I was flattered that he trusted me so much.

During these years I also managed to fit in many weeks working for a local firm of solicitors with whom I subsequently underwent Articles (now called a training contract). There was a novel work tradition called a lunch break in those heady days and most lunchtimes we would go next door to the estate agent's to play Mahjong (a brief glimpse into a bygone age!). We have a wonderful Mahjong set at home gathering dust because the game's popularity (outside the Chinese community) has dwindled over the years.

But perhaps the most entertaining moments of holiday employment were during my time spent working for the Prudential Assurance Company in Reading, which I did for a few weeks in the summers of 1980 and 1981 after my second and third years at Kingston. It was a huge local employer and many went on to work at "The Pru" after leaving school. My job – tea lady. My uniform – a fetching little number: brown dress with brown and white frilly check pinny and matching headband.

Early morning saw me preparing and wrapping sandwiches and salads for the cold shelf, lunchtimes serving behind the counter, while in late afternoon I would be found with my head in commercial ovens, cleaning vigorously. *Elf and Safety* were not in evidence then, so I lost count of the number of times I burned my hands and forearms.

The real fun came mid-morning and mid-afternoon when I toured the building with my tea trolley, providing refreshment to the hard-working employees.

Firstly, I would have to load my trolley in the kitchen. On the top would be the hot water urn with saucers piled up next to it and underneath the cups and biscuits. The routine was to stop my trolley at certain points along the route, staff would line up alongside and collect a saucer and biscuits. I would pick up a cup, pour the drink, hand it to the punter and take payment.

The most amusing stop on my route was in a large open-plan office affectionately known as the Punch Room. It was so-called because it housed row upon row of young women who spent their days in front of bulky VDUs with word processors, "punching in" information long before Microsoft Word came

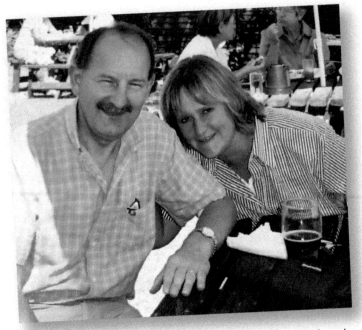

Vinny and I enjoying lunch in a break from my first treatment for cancer in July 2004

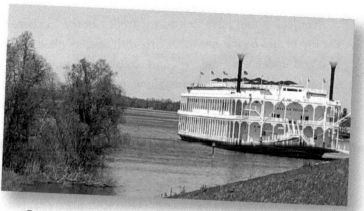

Our mode of conveyance on the Mississippi between Memphis and New Orleans in April 2019

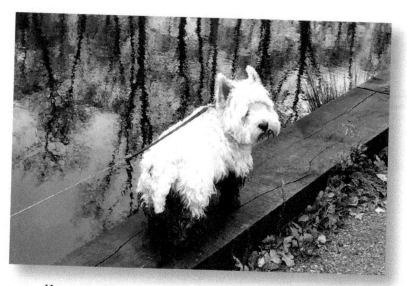

Harvey models his designer 'Mud' boots on the Basingstoke Canal in December 2018

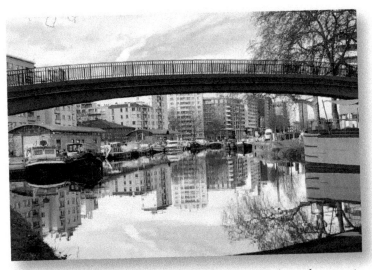

The Canal du Midi in Toulouse. The towpath formed our route to the Stade Ernest-Wallon Stadium for a Bath rugby match in January 2019

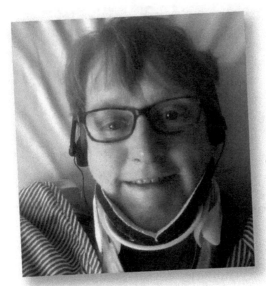

Sporting my neck brace for the first time during my stay at Basingstoke Hospital in March 2020

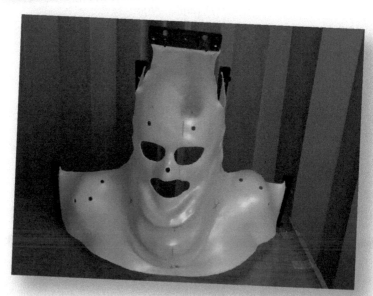

My tailor made radiotherapy mask. March 2020

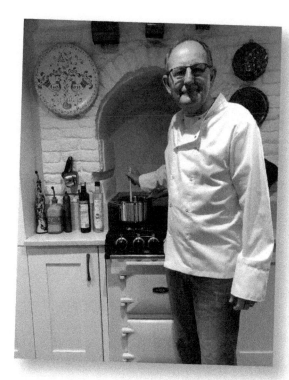

Vinny the Pinny creating his Vogg Victuals in March 2020

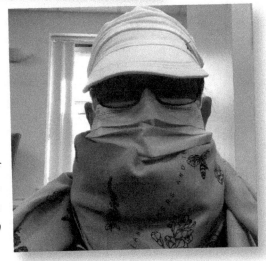

Playing the role of urban guerilla at the Shunting Shed in May 2020

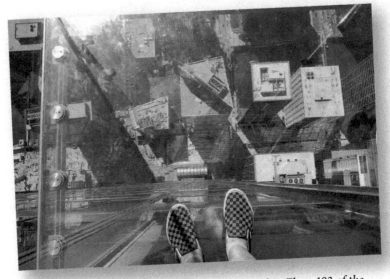

Testing my basophobia to the limit on The Ledge. Floor 103 of the Willis Tower, Chicago. August 2012

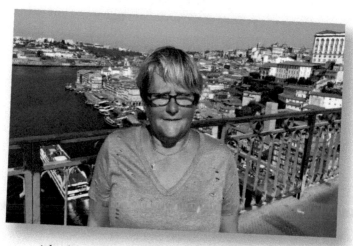

A bridge too far judging from the fear on my face! Luis I Bridge, Porto. August 2018

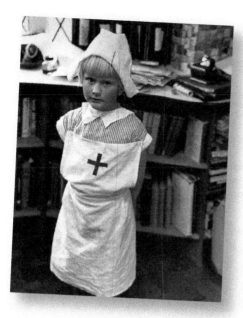

My first shot at testing career choices at the age of five. 1965

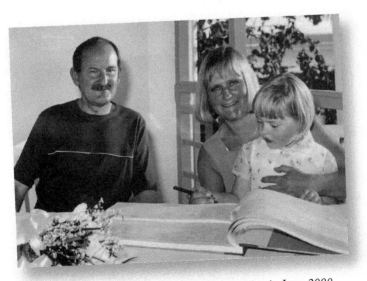

Signing the marriage register in Mauritius in June 2000

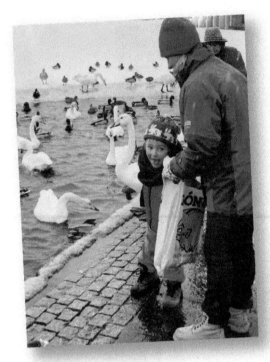

Leah feeding the swans and geese in Reykjavik in February 2001

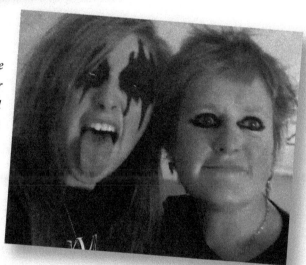

In the zone with Leah for the Black Veil Brides concert at Shepherds Bush in October 2011

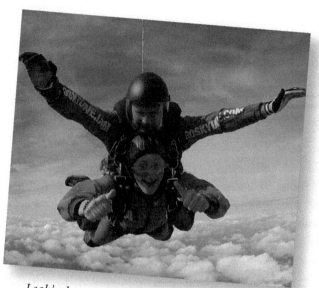

Leah's charity skydive for the Duke of Edinburgh's Diamond Pin Award in 2016

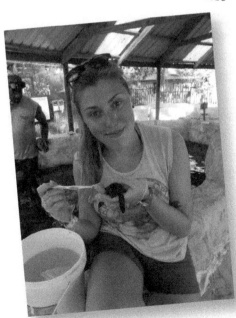

Leah caring for baby turtles while volunteering in Fiji in July 2016

along. It was not the most intellectually demanding task that the Prudential had to offer and, sadly, the Punch Room operators were rather looked-down-upon by employees in other sections. Consequently, they in turn enjoyed looking down on me, given my position on the lowest rung of the ladder.

The Punch Room was so vast that I had to make three stops within the room to allow them all to have their regulation breaks. They partook of coffee in the morning and tea in the afternoon, housed in tiny breakout areas containing soft seating. This ensured they did not have to leave the Punch Room, even during breaks.

On my first day I clattered through the swing doors, using the trolley to push them open, to be met by the initial cohort. I politely asked if this was where I stopped, only for one to sneeringly respond, "No – there," pointing to a spot six inches further on. *Don't try and take me on,* I thought.

Thereafter it became a bit of a game. Every day they would try and add up the cost of various cups of tea/coffee and packets of biscuits, to no avail, and every day they failed to understand how I managed the sums so much more quickly. On days when I was feeling particularly mischievous, I would load the saucers on the opposite side of the urn. I would smile as I watched them struggle to lean across and collect a saucer rather than work out it might be easier to queue on the other side. Such little amusements in a humdrum day!

Having completed the route, I would then wait in a lobby area by the lifts, having my own cuppa and counting the money before taking the reverse route to collect the empties and return to the kitchen.

On my last day of my second year, I was minding my own

business, drinking my coffee and counting the money, when a smarmy manager sidled up to me. The conversation went thus:

Mr Greaseball: *"Hello, darling, I don't think we've met."*

Me: *"No, sir, I don't think we have."*

Mr Greaseball: *(getting ever closer and invading my personal space) "And have you been here long?"*

Me: *"Well, sir, this is my second year but it also happens to be my last day."*

Mr Greaseball: *(almost salivating) "Oh yes, and what are you going to be doing?"*

Me: *"I've just finished my law degree and I'm off to the Guildford College of Law to complete my Solicitor's Final Exams."*

Mr Greaseball, colour draining from his face, could not exit my personal space fast enough and scurried back to his office like the weasel that he was!

Looking back, I do think that undertaking part-time jobs of that nature provided valuable workplace insights and life skills before launching head first into permanent careers. But the most important lesson I learned was that you do need a strong sense of humour to be able to cope with what is thrown at you, both at the time and in later life.

Having completed my education at Kingston and the Guildford College of Law, I then entered the world of full-time employment and, after two years of Articles, was admitted to the roll of solicitors in October 1984. I have been qualified as such for over thirty-five years and have been fortunate enough to have had, overall, a thoroughly enjoyable career, much of it based as a criminal defence lawyer in the counties of Hampshire and Surrey.

Taking the first tentative steps on my chosen career path filled me with a heady mixture of excitement and awe. I knew straightaway that I had made the right choice and that this was going to be the life for me.

6

Duty Cutie

At one of my local magistrates' courts, Aldershot, in the Eighties and Nineties, one of the regular magistrates was known as the Nodding Magistrate or sometimes the Smiling Assassin. He would pay close attention to an advocate making a bail application, nodding sagely and earnestly throughout as if he was agreeing with every word, then burst the bubble of confidence by saying, "Remand in custody."

Despite this, I liked him; you always knew where you stood with him. I recall one Saturday morning when I was on the rota as duty solicitor. As I entered the building, he was emerging from the court office. He greeted me with words that I have never forgotten (and which continue to make me smile) – "Good Morning, Issy. Are you today's Duty Cutie?" While I appreciate that, in this day and age, such an address might be thought of as offensive, sexist and patronising, back then it was meant as nothing more than an innocent endearment. I certainly did not feel threatened or insulted.

So how did I become a duty solicitor? To answer that question, I have to return to the autumn of 1974 when I was fourteen and in my fourth year (known these days as Year 10). At that time, work experience was very much an *ad hoc* event, organised by individual schools speaking with local businesses. A Wokingham solicitor came into school to provide a career talk and made the offer of some half-term experience, which I accepted. To be frank, looking at fusty law books in a draughty timber-framed medieval office building was not my idea of fun. I bunked off before the end of the week but not before a recently qualified assistant solicitor had taken me to the Royal Courts of Justice in central London, and Slough Magistrates' Court in Berkshire.

In the former I was fascinated by the multitude of rooms and courts found in the labyrinthine corridors of the Gothic Revival building and transfixed by the goings-on in the Bear Gardens, more of which later.

In contrast, Slough Magistrates' Court was a boring Sixties building that has not changed since that first visit over forty years ago. But there was something about the grittiness of the place and the work conducted there. No doubt influenced by the sense of injustice experienced in class as a young child, I became hooked and, from then on, I wanted to be a criminal lawyer.

Back then, in the late Seventies, this necessitated obtaining a university degree followed by postgraduate study for professional exams. I took the route of a law degree with one postgraduate year but there was also the option of a non-law degree followed by two postgraduate years.

The whole university application process, in an era when there were no open days, coaching, mentoring or personal statements, really was quite a daunting experience (as was the transition straight into employment for those not choosing or able to enter further education on a full-time basis).

Oxford was my first choice, but coming from a state grammar school with no real history of Oxbridge success, I had no idea of what to expect. I passed the entrance exam and was called for interview. I had to go up the night before to dine. I was well looked-after by some Philosophy, Politics and

Economics (PPE) students but, for a naive seventeen-year-old from the Wokingham outback, it was all rather surreal. I was given an article on recidivism to read, and forty minutes of the forty-five-minute-long interview was spent discussing it. Not being an ardent recidivism scholar, it came as no surprise that the feedback to school indicated that I was less than forthcoming at interview!

My other choices were Bristol, Exeter, University College London and Liverpool. Because we were left to fend for ourselves, and not understanding the process, I firmly, rather than provisionally, accepted an offer from UCL. Thereafter I immediately received rejections from all of the others. I did not then achieve the grades needed for UCL. Having been very successful in my O levels, I had not appreciated the extent of the jump up to A levels (or to the S level I studied for in German) and failed to put in sufficient effort, preferring to head off to the squash court or golf course.

I went through clearing and was offered a place at Goldsmiths College, now known as Goldsmiths, University of London, but to read history. Despite this, I really wanted to study law so opted to take a place I had been offered at Kingston Polytechnic. That proved, both at the time and later in life, to be the best choice I could possibly have made.

Once at Kingston I learned that it was, at the time, regarded as the third best law school in the country after Cambridge and Birmingham Universities. The degree was very practical in focus and set me in good stead. More importantly, I met some great people and had a whale of a time. We did not have that many hours of formal tuition but I still managed to miss some lectures because of rugby or squash commitments, or through carrying on with a game of darts or table football in the student union bar.

The highlight of the whole Kingston Poly social calendar was the Law Society annual pantomime. We had great fun writing and performing in them – for instance, one year we did *Peter Pan* as a version of *Grease*. But those years were the pinnacle of my acting and playwriting careers!

From Kingston I went on to the Guildford College of Law to study for my professional exams. Once there I realised the huge benefit of having a degree from Kingston. We fared so much better than the Oxbridge graduates who had tended to major on the theoretical and academic.

So, while destiny may not have taken me down the path I had intended, the outcome nevertheless proved far more satisfying and rewarding. This experience turned me into something of a fatalist, in the sense that the opportunities that have presented themselves in life may not have been the ones I had planned or expected, but embracing them fully and energetically has always produced positive results.

Having completed my academic studies in 1982, I then commenced two years of practical training, employed as an articled clerk (now called trainee solicitor) with a firm of solicitors operating from offices in East Sheen, Richmond and Wokingham. As well as learning the practicalities of the law, I was also expected to muck in with the junior administrative staff, tasks that I had absolutely no objection to carrying out. It demonstrated that I was not above myself and helped foster good office relationships. I remember happily trotting around Richmond Green and the High Street at the end of each day, delivering local post to other solicitors and estate agents.

Another administrative duty was to provide relief coverage as a telephonist at lunchtimes. The firm owned a really old-fashioned switchboard, which required incoming calls to be connected with intended recipients by inserting cable jacks into the appropriate sockets and flicking switches – "You're though now!" How times have changed in less than forty years.

When describing my administrative duties to Vinny he explained that he went through a similar induction process when he joined the Ministry of Defence in Bath way back in 1969. As the most junior newbie in the office, he was allocated all of those menial tasks that nobody else would do, including making the tea and coffee. His predecessor taught him the drill, including who had what in which cup and how to clean up afterwards. After wiping everything down she finished with a flourish. "If there is anybody you don't particularly like," she said, "such as Claude in my case, you just squeeze the dishcloth into their cup like this." His first bit of on-the-job training, but his first refusal to follow a mentor's advice!

My professional duties during my Articles were many and varied. I thought I had struck it lucky very early on when I discovered that one of the firm's clients was a large brewery. At the time the brewery decided to sell off a substantial number of its tied properties at auction, and one of my tasks during my conveyancing training was to prepare the necessary legal packs (the documents you must always read as they advise on BBC's *Homes Under the Hammer*). I also assisted prospective purchasers at the auctions that were held at a central London hotel – with lunch provided; most propitious for an impecunious trainee!

Opportunities to undertake advocacy were limited during Articles as it is necessary to be qualified to have full rights of audience in open court. I did appear in interim hearings held in chambers, but my most terrifying experience was in the Bear Garden in the Royal Courts of Justice. In simplistic terms, the Bear Garden is where parties go to request an order and is usually frequented by trainees cutting their advocacy teeth. Everyone attends together to await their turn and the Masters (judges) are fearsome. It was given its name when Queen Victoria paid a visit to the Royal Courts of Justice following its opening and, on hearing the cacophony from the open area, likened it to a garden of bears.

Once qualified as a solicitor I was able to appear regularly in the magistrate's court. My first guilty plea was for a youth who had stolen a pair of trainers. My first not-guilty trial was for a young girl accused of damaging a street bollard in Aldershot town centre. I was so nervous, and very much appreciated the assistance given to me by older hands. Consequently, I have always tried to assist the newly qualified who find themselves in a similar situation.

Ever since those early cases my career has been focused entirely on criminal law. More particularly I took the conscious decision to work as a defence lawyer rather than a prosecutor, apart from a six-month period in 1989 when I joined the Crown Prosecution Service (CPS) to view life from the other side of the professional fence. Apart from that valuable six-month period, I have spent my entire career defending clients in the criminal courts within both the civilian and military jurisdictions.

Contrary to popular belief, influenced by some media misreporting, the work of a criminal defence lawyer is not particularly well remunerated considering the qualifications, degree of training and professional status required. The legal aid rates paid in respect of clients who are publicly funded, who represent the vast majority, have not been increased for around twenty-five years and, in some categories, have actually been reduced. In 2020 a fully qualified and well-established criminal defence lawyer would be doing well to earn between £35,000 and £40,000 per annum. But those solicitors who elect to specialise in the criminal law invariably do so out of a sense of vocation, including the delivery of a justice system that is fair and open to all, rather than any pecuniary considerations. I would certainly put myself in that bracket, having been driven by a clear sense of justice and the importance of fair play from my early classroom experience.

The majority of defence solicitors also become duty solicitors as I did in 1986, following the inception of the duty scheme that year. As such I have been a frequent visitor to police stations to assist clients on arrest or when invited for voluntary interview. It is possible to be called out at any time during each twelve-hour day or night duty period, and for any alleged type of crime, ranging from shoplifting to murder. If the services of the duty solicitor are required because the arrested person wishes to be represented but does not have their own nominated solicitor, the police custody staff will contact a call centre who in turn contact the rota solicitor, with each solicitor having their own PIN. I am now such an old hand that mine is in the 400s, whereas newly qualified duty solicitors today will have a PIN in the 15000s.

As well as being a police station duty solicitor I am a court duty solicitor, whose role is to look after eligible unrepresented defendants.

Throughout my long and rewarding career, I have only worked with seven firms of solicitors plus the CPS. When thinking about job interviews for those positions, I have to say that the informality and, indeed, irregularity of the vast majority of them would be regarded as unacceptable in today's more regulated and politically correct world.

I was never interviewed *per se* by the firm with whom I did my Articles – or training contract in today's parlance – principally because I had worked for them while studying for my law degree. I was fortunate enough to have secured paid work experience while studying as a result of writing around offering my services to a number of local firms. I was awarded the work experience position following a positive response to one of my letters and a chat in a nearby pub with one of the firm's partners. At the completion of my Articles, I was offered a post with the firm as a qualified solicitor, but I decided that it would be better for my career to move on. I therefore prepared for, what I thought, would be my first set of formal job interviews as I embarked on my legal career in earnest.

I recall being interviewed by a small, but upmarket firm of solicitors in Conduit Street, in the Mayfair area of London. The office was very flash with a fountain in the foyer. The interview went well until I raised the thorny issue of salary. I received a sneered response, "Well, you have come from the provinces." I would not be accepting a job offer here, I resolved immediately!

The first solicitor's job I took was in Fleet, Hampshire in 1984. I was interviewed by the senior criminal partner, Mike, who kindly ran me back to the station. A short while later, while still waiting for my train, I saw him running over the bridge waving the umbrella that I had left in his office. *Oh no, I have blown this one*, I thought. But I had not and I stayed for four years, being made a salaried partner after eighteen months.

Six months into the job the senior partner of another local firm invited me for a glass of wine after court one day. It did not take long for me to realise that he was actually interviewing me. Not having much regard for either his approach or firm I diplomatically extricated myself from the situation.

On relating the event to Mike, he was furious. The same solicitor had poached my predecessor, hence my appointment.

After several years in Fleet, I decided it was time for a change. Word got out on the local legal network and I received a call from the Branch Crown Prosecutor in Basingstoke. Could I start at the CPS on the following Monday? And I did. I thought it would be good for me to see life from a different professional perspective.

After six months, and with a reference from the then Chief Crown Prosecutor of Dorset and Hampshire, I applied for a Senior Crown Prosecutor's position. I would have stayed with the CPS had I secured the post, but without interview, I was offered a basic Crown Prosecutor role instead. Appalled at the lack of due and fair process, I thought, *Stuff that, I'm heading back to the dark side*. This despite the restrictive covenant imposed by my previous employer in Fleet not to work within their catchment area for a period of two years. I did, however, enjoy my six months as a prosecutor and learned a great deal in the process.

A round of eclectic interviews and offers ensued. There was an in-house position at the RSPCA but that was too political for me. Another in-house position emerged at British Telecom in the East End of London, but I did not fancy the commute. At a firm in Basingstoke the interviewer insisted on speaking to me in German for reasons that remain obscure. A firm in Southampton enclosed a £1,000 golden handshake cheque in their offer letter with the comment that encashment would be deemed as acceptance of the job. I ripped up the cheque and declined the offer, pointing out that I did not operate like that.

I had virtually resolved to accept the offer of a job in Petersfield, Hampshire, when another became available in Epsom, Surrey. On the weekend prior to the interview, having overimbibed at a party, I twisted my ankle. The senior criminal partner roared with laughter at my very honest explanation for hobbling into the interview and I got the job without further ado

Having served my two-year exclusion from the Fleet area, I signed up with an agency and, lo and behold, was told that an Aldershot firm was very interested in my CV, initially provided anonymously by the agency. On ascertaining that the firm was Tanner and Taylor (T & T), who I knew from my earlier experience in the area, I indicated that I was happy for my name to go forward.

The next day I received a call from the then senior partner, Ian, which went as follows:

Ian: *"Why the %^*# didn't you ring me direct? Now I've got to pay an agency fee!"*
Me: *"Oh, I've got the job then, have I? Thanks."*
Ian: *"When can you start?"*

By the time I left T&T nineteen years later I was the Senior Criminal Partner and Personnel Partner with a staff of over sixty. However, in the end I had come to the conclusion that there was too much administration for my liking and not enough lawyering.

From 2009 I had six very happy years with Coomber Rich in Basingstoke. The interview with Jo Coomber consisted of me swivelling round on a reception chair in her offices, a chat in our summer house, then Vinny and I having a pleasant dinner at Jo's house one Saturday evening.

After a short spell working from home on a project with a barristers' chambers in London (for which no interview was involved), I took up my current consultancy position with Levales in Ash Vale, Hampshire, following a very agreeable lunch with their managing partner, Drew, in September 2017. They are a great team and I have thoroughly enjoyed my time working with them.

So, a quick canter through my career has confirmed that the majority of my moves have been based on informal chats and nods rather than properly conducted interviews. I have, however, been subjected to one modern-day structured interview, which proved both gruelling and satisfying in equal measure.

This took place in 2015 at a time when tendering proposals for legal aid contracts were threatening the legal defence world as we knew it, with the very real prospect of many firms going to the wall. I applied for a job as a qualified caseworker at the Court of Appeal preparing case papers for their Lords Justices. The work would have been demanding but extremely interesting. Having completed a very detailed application form, along with my very first experience of psychometric testing, I was astonished to be shortlisted for an interview. It consisted of firstly sitting a forty-five-minute paper, commenting on three legal problems, immediately followed by a similar length face-to-face grilling by a panel of three.

You cannot imagine my reaction when I was advised that I had only just been pipped at the post, effectively coming second in a national recruitment drive for a Court of Appeal lawyer. They decided to hold matters open for twelve months so that if another position became available in that time, I could be appointed without further interview. In the event, another position did not become available, but I have to admit that I was not disappointed. It avoided having to make what would have been an incredibly difficult decision about changing my work-life balance just as I was approaching the age of fifty-five, particularly given the need to commute. But it was hugely satisfying to have been able to master modern-day interview techniques, after thirty years of rather less robust practices, and outpoint so many young guns in the process!

Covid-19 created the inevitable use of virtual courts and police station interviews, with much greater dependency on technology. This all came into play while I was shielding due to cancer treatment. The transition to a more technologically based approach has clear potential benefits, and is long overdue, but I have to say that I would have missed the closer, interpersonal engagement that will be lost as a result had my condition allowed me to return to full time practice.

Although it is doubtful that I would have retired at this juncture had cancer and a related fractured neck not intervened, the impact of Covid-19 has nevertheless helped ease my decision to hang up my wig and gown and withdraw gracefully. In doing so I can now consign my duty-cutie experiences to memory or to the next chapter in the case of the more unusual and noteworthy.

7

Crime Pays (But Only Just)

As a criminal defence lawyer, I represented clients from a wide range of backgrounds accused of every conceivable type of crime from shoplifting to murder across England and Wales and, in the case of military clients, at bases overseas. In doing so I inevitably saw a very broad spectrum of life. I also witnessed every form of human emotion along the way. A number of cases stand out in my mind because they were particularly unusual, sad, complex, brutal, challenging or surreal, or gave rise to moments of humour, whether intended or otherwise. In sharing my recollections of some of these more notable cases I should first like to reassure that I have been careful not to breach any client confidentiality. What follows reflects matters that were aired in open court, and are therefore already in the public domain, or are of a peripheral nature only.

Before stepping into my mental locker room of indelible cases, I think it might be helpful to explain the principal role of a defence lawyer and the responsibility he or she has towards their client.

To begin at a basic level, the job of the defence lawyer is to explain to the client the strengths and weaknesses of the case against them, outline the consequences of pleading guilty or not guilty and represent them in their best possible interests according to their response to the allegations that have been made.

Clearly there are cases when the evidence is weak, or

where the defence has in its possession evidence to refute the prosecution case, in which circumstances a trial is the appropriate course of action. There are also occasions when those charged with an offence will find that the strength of evidence against them is overwhelming but they continue to deny guilt despite the incredulity of their alibi or explanation. In such an event the defence lawyer can do little more than accept the client's instructions and do their very best for them in the circumstances that prevail. I will expand on the reasons for this a little later.

In reality, when the evidence against them is strong and fully explained, a high proportion of clients plead guilty accordingly. Amongst this cadre are those, often first-time offenders, who have been involved in a drunken brawl and have no recollection of the event. The absence of recollection often equates to a denial – until CCTV footage is shown. The standard sequence of events prior to police interview in such cases runs something like this.

Me: "Now you've been arrested because, it is said, you have punched and kicked the complainant outside the Emporium in Fleet town centre."

Mr Denial: "No, no way. I wouldn't do that. I swear on my baby daughter's life I didn't do it."

Me: "Well, there is CCTV evidence. Let's watch it.

(CCTV watched together – shows Mr Denial knocking seven bells out of the complainant.)

Mr Denial: (head in hands) "Oh my God. Oh no. I can't believe it."

During the first Covid-19 lockdown in 2020 the Prime Minister's special adviser, Dominic Cummings, was famously outed for not only travelling 250 miles to County Durham but, while there, being spotted driving to Barnard Castle. His explanation was that he was testing his eyesight. Not surprisingly that produced much mirth on social media given the dubious credibility of such an explanation, including an ironic tweet from *The Secret Barrister* announcing that

```
today's alleged shoplifter was going to be a swift
guilty plea but may be worth a trial on the basis he
was testing the capacity of his pockets ...
```

The reference in that tweet to alleged shoplifting immediately brought to mind a trial very early on in my career at Coventry Magistrates' Court. My client had purchased a pair of sandals at a hypermarket on the outskirts of Reading. She had the sandals in her bag when she travelled to Coventry with her daughter for a swimming competition. (Little did I realise that, twenty years later, I too would be travelling long distances to support my daughter at national swimming competitions!)

While in a store in Coventry, my client spotted an identical pair of sandals at a much cheaper price. She took her own sandals out of her bag to make a comparison before placing them back in her bag. Unfortunately, the store detective only spotted the act of replacement and jumped to the immediate, and mistaken, conclusion that my client was in the act of stealing a pair of sandals from the store shelves.

The store detective, in her evidence, explained that she had followed my client into the ladies' toilet where she observed my client removing other items from her bag so that she could "hide" the sandals at the bottom.

My client did, indeed, accept that she had visited the toilet and, in looking for something in her bag, had taken items out. When she repacked her bag, the sandals she had bought in Reading had ended up at the bottom. But this action of removing and replacing items had taken place in the cubicle while she was actually sitting on the toilet.

The store detective had to accept in cross-examination that the only way she had been able to observe my client's actions was by getting down on her hands and knees in the next-door cubicle and looking under the dividing wall! The magistrates were so appalled by this invasion of privacy that they instantly acquitted my client without the need for me to address them on the evidence supporting the purchase in Reading.

Another case that gave rise to some amusing exchanges involved a football match many years ago when all weekend matches kicked off at 3.00 p.m. on a Saturday afternoon and finished at around 4.45 p.m., and district judges in the magistrates' court were called stipendiary magistrates (or stipes for short).

I was representing three lads, Chelsea supporters, who were charged with throwing coins on to the pitch from The Shed at Stamford Bridge during a derby game against Spurs. They were very respectable, articulate lads who were adamant that they had done nothing wrong and had simply been pulled out of the crowd before the end of the game by unnecessarily aggressive police officers, including one in particular – PC Bumptious, a Spurs supporter.

He had been abusive to them and very unprofessional, due

to the rivalry between opposing supporters, while transporting them in the meat wagon back to the police station.

I had watched the relevant CCTV footage, a short passage, in my office with the lads before the trial. It took the four of us some considerable time, and many replays, to finally pick them out in the middle of The Shed. There was certainly no evidence of coin-throwing. PC Bumptious had been on duty pitch-side at the juncture of The Shed and a neighbouring stand, some considerable distance away.

The day of the trial came and, naturally, the prosecution star witness was PC Bumptious. As he came into the witness box it was clearly evident that his whole assessment of self-worth and importance was in inverse proportion to his inherent levels of integrity and competence. His manner was aggressive, chest puffed out, his body language suggestive of his overriding belief that his evidence would be accepted whether truthful or not. That was a bad mistake – it is a particular joy for a criminal defence advocate to demonstrably catch out a police officer being economical with the truth while in the witness box.

He gave his evidence in anticipated obnoxious style. My cross-examination of him went something like this.

Me: "Officer, please can we watch the CCTV." (CCTV played.)

Stipe Grumpy: "Why are we watching this – it doesn't show anything."

Me: "Exactly, sir, but if I may be allowed to continue. Officer, please pick out my clients on the screen."

PC Bumptious: (peers at the screen) "I'm afraid I can't do so on this small screen."

Me: "So let me understand this. You are unable to pick them out from the CCTV of the relevant section of the crowd but, on the day, you were able to locate and pick them out in the stand from your physical position a considerable distance away. Is that correct?"

PC Bumptious: (beginning to falter and failing to answer the question) "I saw them throwing coins."

Me: "You're a Spurs supporter, aren't you?"

PC Bumptious: "Yes." (By throwing him a googly he had answered the question before giving thought as to why I was asking it.)

Stipe Grumpy: "What's wrong with being a Spurs fan? I am."

Me: "Absolutely nothing wrong with that, sir, but if I may be allowed to continue. Officer, you didn't see my clients throwing coins at all. You just wanted to arrest Chelsea fans. You were then abusive to them in the van on the way to the police station, which is how they knew you were a Spurs supporter."

PC Bumptious: (now very defensive) "That's not true. They must have heard me on the radio asking my mates for the result."

Me: "Officer. It was 4.40 p.m. The game hadn't finished, had it?"

PC Bumptious: (crestfallen and shaking, fails to answer)

Me: (observing the cross-examination rule of quitting while ahead) "No further questions."

My clients gave evidence impeccably and it was then time for my closing speech. I rose to my feet expecting to do battle with the Spurs-supporting stipe.

Me: "Sir—"
Stipe Grumpy: (interrupting) "No need to address me.
Not Guilty."
Me: (mentally punching the air) "Thank you, sir."

PC Bumptious skulked out of court with his tail between his legs, having had to listen to the stipe pass adverse comment on the veracity of the prosecution evidence. I learned a lot that day. I was only about three or four years qualified and was still at the stage when I thought cross-examination needed to be conducted by an aggressive Rottweiler. But this time I had achieved my goal by being polite, restrained and targeted.

I later became involved in another football-related trial at Aldershot Magistrates' Court that arose out of events on 12 September 1987 when Aldershot FC, then in the old Division Three, were at home to Brighton and Hove Albion. A large crowd was expected and, sure enough, the ground was full to capacity before kick-off. In those days, due to frequent violence between opposing fans, a "sterile area" was created in the middle of the East Terrace, which was heavily policed. Aldershot lost 1-4 and the mood turned ugly. Shots fans were upset by the taunting directed towards them by the Seagulls and, despite the police presence, violence broke out.

Apart from the fans themselves, the main protagonists were Chief Inspector Hapless, PC Thumper and PC Reckless with his police dog, Gnasher.

I was on the rota as a duty solicitor on the day in question and my knowledge of the rivalry between Aldershot and Brighton fans suggested that it was going to be busy. I was not disappointed! I was called out to represent five Seagulls fans.

They and a number of Shots fans were charged with a variety of offences, including violent disorder, a then relatively new offence under the 1984 Public Order Act that came into force in January 1986. Not knowing what to expect, the magistrates agreed to hold the trial at Aldershot Magistrates' Court – they never did so again and violent disorder cases always now go to the Crown Court.

So, there we were, ready to start a trial that was to last eight days. Very early on we had a site visit. Imagine the magistrates picking over the East Terrace at the Recreation Ground, Aldershot, to glean an understanding of the purpose of a sterile area and its operation!

One of my clients, Mr Lucksout, was charged with assaulting PC Thumper and resisting arrest. During the incident Mr Lucksout sustained a nasty injury to his mouth, losing some teeth into the bargain. PC Thumper, in his statement, said this had happened while Mr Lucksout was on the ground resisting arrest. Mr Lucksout maintained it had happened when PC Thumper had slammed his face against a windowsill, and expert medical evidence supported my client's account.

Cross-examination of PC Thumper went something like this.

Me: *"You've seen the medical evidence. It doesn't support your account."*

PC Thumper: *"Well, I've just remembered that he hit*

his face on the wall before ending up on the floor."
    *Me: "In which case he'd have injuries to his chin and
nose, which he hasn't."*
    PC Thumper: (silent, shifting, blushing)
    Result: Acquittal.

Another of my clients was charged with assaulting Chief
Inspector Hapless by causing him to sustain a broken wrist.
The chief inspector was clearly in the thick of it and trying to
arrest my client. In cross-examination PC Reckless admitted
that, out of concern that the chief inspector was out of his depth
by being involved in frontline policing, he had waded in with
Gnasher at his side and truncheon waving. Unfortunately, his
truncheon came into contact with the chief inspector's wrist,
causing the break in true Keystone Cops style.

The prosecutor and I stood there literally open-mouthed.
While PC Reckless had to be given credit for his honesty, it was
astonishing that the true position had not been made known
sooner and that the prosecution of my client had reached trial
stage. Not surprisingly he was also acquitted.

Although there had, undoubtedly, been disorder that day,
the police did not cover themselves in glory in their anxiety to
secure convictions. But we are talking over thirty years ago and
a lot has happened since then in terms of police accountability!

Another serious offence under the Public Order Act is riot.
While working in Epsom I acted for three brothers, local ne'er-
do-wells but good clients! One Friday night they and four mates
went across to a pub in Wallington, Surrey. Unsurprisingly
there was a massive punch-up. As a result, they and one local

Wallington lad ended up at Guildford Crown Court on trial for riot. I acted for all eight but, through the local lad, garnered twenty-four defence witnesses.

The general consensus of opinion was that, while the Epsom lads were looking for trouble, the real problem was caused by the arrival of the Met Police. The development of events thereafter was rather farcical.

We knew from the radio reports that when the shout went out for police assistance, it was picked up by the Territorial Support Group (TSG), which, at the time, had a reputation for a rather over-zealous approach.

The TSG were looking for some action that night and came flying across South London before bursting into the pub with truncheons waving. The unit consisted of one inspector, one sergeant and seven PCs. It was obvious from the radio reports that they decided *en route* that the incident they were heading towards was a riot, so ensured that they arrested twelve people, the number needed for a riot charge under the Public Order Act. This included a female who sat up front in the unit paddy wagon with the inspector, giving directions to Epsom Police Station. On arrival she was de-arrested along with three others, leaving the eight who I then represented.

Once at Epsom Police Station matters for the police went from bad to worse. Their woes while there emerged from cross-examination during the trial. Firstly, the TSG sergeant took over as custody sergeant in the cells at Epsom, which is completely against the rules. Secondly, he got the whole TSG unit together to write up their statements, including the use of each defendant's name when describing their alleged part in the incident.

Unfortunately for the police officers, the judge ruled that as they did not know the defendants, their names must have been obtained from their own sergeant during the booking-in process, which thus amounted to hearsay evidence and were therefore inadmissible. As a consequence, in evidence they were only permitted to use physical descriptions, none of which they had managed to record in any detail.

It transpired from the resultant farce that one of my clients was supposedly being booked into custody at the very time he was receiving treatment in A&E. Another miraculously appeared to have removed his singlet while lying handcuffed on the floor of the unit paddy wagon. I still remember the vehicle's call sign, E515, and it had to be brought to court for the jury to inspect.

The inspector denied, when asked, the presence of a female. But he had obviously failed to brief his PCs, one of whom, when asked the same question, replied, "Oh, you mean the one that gave us directions to the police station."

At the outset of the prosecution case the jury were looking daggers at the defendants in the dock. As the days passed those looks turned to ones of humour and sympathy. Eventually, the judge turned to prosecuting counsel and, in a slightly exasperated tone, asked him if he wanted to continue.

The next morning the CPS finally threw in the towel and the defendants were acquitted.

As can be seen from the narration of this case, my role as a criminal defence solicitor is not confined to court advocacy. I spend as much time, if not more, representing clients in the police station. One such example involved a client arrested for murder, who was clearly suffering from severe mental health issues. Three times I opined to the custody sergeant that my client was not fit to be interviewed, and three times the police surgeon said he was.

Whether the custody sergeant agreed with me or was simply mocking me I do not know, but he directed that an appropriate adult (a suitable person whose role is to aid communication between the detainee and the police) should be present in interview.

To my dismay, a rather timid community psychiatric nurse turned up, who did not match the calibre of your average CPN.

The police interview began and the client was happy to talk freely. It would not be appropriate for me to recite the facts, save to say that the account given could have been used as the script for a remake of *Silence of the Lambs*. It was obvious that the interviewing officers did not believe the account and stated they would be back later for further interviews. They returned in under an hour, white as sheets, to charge him with murder.

On enquiring about the sudden change of strategy, I was advised that evidence had been found at the scene of crime to support the client's gruesome account.

The next day Mr Timid rang me to offer counselling. Well, you can imagine my response to that!!

As an afterthought to this case, I recall treating myself to a pamper week at Champneys Health Spa in the mid-Eighties. While there I was told that the maid had gone into Anthony Hopkins's room to clean, not realising that he was still in the shower. Apparently, he emerged, hair slicked back, at which the maid ran screaming from the room. It took some considerable time to convince her that she had not just encountered Hannibal Lecter!

In particularly serious cases, the police may need more time for questioning than is initially allowed by the legislation, so they need to apply to the local magistrates' court for further time.

Many years ago, a client had been arrested in relation to an historical, but serious, allegation and was being interviewed in Alton Police Station. The police decided that they needed to make an application for further time, which required us all to travel to Aldershot Magistrates' Court, some eight miles away.

We all went in a police transit van, the two CID officers up front in the driver and passenger seat, with my client and me in the back. It was all very friendly and my client was not even handcuffed. I have to say it is a situation that simply would not be permitted today.

On approaching a roundabout on the Farnham bypass, the traffic lights turned to red. It was clear that the driver of the vehicle in front of us was intending to carry on through the lights. At the last minute she must have realised that there was a large police vehicle looming up behind her and she slammed on the anchors. Our CID driver did exactly the same and how we did not go into the back of her I will never know. But, as a result, my client and I ended up in a heap together on the floor of the van, fortunately without injury.

I am pleased to report that after the magistrates granted further time, we returned to Alton without incident. Subsequently no further action was taken against my client.

I mentioned that my career as a defence lawyer was interrupted in 1989 by a brief, six-month stint with the CPS. In many ways, it was probably the best time to have had some experience of life from a prosecutor's perspective. There did not seem to be any significant funding issues in those days and few top-down constraints from senior management.

As a basic Crown Prosecutor, I was given a lot of discretion over my decision-making. It was great to be able to use my defence experience to spot potential deficiencies in a police file, and requisition action or material to fill the gaps to enable the prosecution to move forward.

By necessarily working 8 a.m. to 6 p.m. I earned two hours' overtime each day – a reward for working beyond conditioned hours that was then more common than it is today! At the start of each week the office staff would place all files requiring attention on a long table under signs denoting type of action, and these were refreshed on a daily basis. I made it my own target to ensure that the table was empty at the end of each week, much to the delight of my colleagues!

It was also a time when we still had lunch breaks. No one worried if the afternoon court session was slightly delayed in recommencing as the prosecutors, defence lawyers and court clerks had invariably been lunching together, often in the pub opposite the magistrates' court! Quite unthinkable today, but the camaraderie engendered helped ensure that the business was executed both efficiently and fairly.

Because I had come straight from defence practice in Aldershot Magistrates' Court, I was unable to prosecute in that court. I knew too many of the defendants. My advocacy was therefore in Basingstoke, Andover and Winchester where there was still a magistrates' court housed within the Crown Court building. Believe it or not, despite Winchester being the county town of Hampshire with a Crown Court that covers the whole of the north of the county, it has not had its own magistrates' court for many years.

Because of my ultra-short spiky haircut that I sported at the time I soon became known as The Punk Prosecutor. I think the local criminal clientele thought that they were being clever by insulting me. But I took it as a compliment – at least they knew who I was and I had therefore made some sort of impression.

At that time juveniles moved up to the adult court at the age of seventeen. There was one obnoxious youngster causing such havoc that the ushers had ringed his seventeenth birthday on their calendar, waiting for his first appearance in the adult court to bring him a wake-up call along with a custodial sentence. The problem was that each time he came to court as a juvenile there would be an adjournment to a future date to add an inevitable new case to the growing list of those that remained unresolved.

This was a pattern that repeated itself with monotonous regularity – until his voluminous file landed in my lap. I insisted before the court that all outstanding cases be dealt with forthwith and that any new cases could wait until a future date. A simple ploy you might think, that resulted in the offender being removed from his scenes of crime prior to his seventeenth birthday.

The reward for my diligence was that all future matters relating to the individual would be assigned to me. Twenty years later I discovered that the juvenile's transition into adulthood had not brought any change to his offending behaviour. When I joined a local firm in 2009, I soon discovered that he was one of their clients!

Another fallout from diligence came from thoroughly

researching all the vehicle tachograph regulations ahead of a trial that had been assigned to me. It was a very dry area of law and not particularly attractive to the majority of my colleagues. My reward for being successful at trial was to find that all tacho cases thereafter miraculously found their way to my desk.

I do look back on that short period of my career with fondness, but I am nevertheless glad that I did return to the dark side. And, of course, I brought with me the experience of how the CPS operated. As the pressures upon the CPS have increased over the years and their resources have diminished, I have never lost my sense of empathy for the challenges they face at a personal and organisational level.

When I moved from the CPS to a firm in Epsom in 1989, the local magistrates' court had a warrant office. This was staffed by a sergeant and two PCs who were coming to the end of their careers. They acted as liaison between the court and the police, executing warrants and acting as dock officers among other duties. I got on very well with them and put my £1 a week into their coffee fund for an endless supply of hot drinks.

The situation comedy *'Allo, 'Allo* was big on our TV screens at the time and the warrant office sergeant named court staff, and some regular solicitors, after characters in the programme. As I was still sporting my spiky haircut, I was known as Helga. One iconic episode featured Helga and her silk knickers bearing little swastikas. As my thirtieth birthday approached the warrant officers kept asking me if I was going to wear the knickers with the little swastikas.

I decided to take them by surprise. At the time I had a suit with a wrap-around skirt. I bought a pair of French knickers that looked like shorts and, using a black marker pen, covered them in little swastikas. The morning of my thirtieth birthday arrived and I headed down to court. As soon as I got into the warrant office one of the PCs whisked me up and placed me standing on a chair and asked, "Where are the knickers with the little swastikas?" I was able to simply lift one side of my wrap-around skirt to reveal them without being indecent. The warrant officers fell about with laughter – they thought I was just going to produce something from my pocket.

News spread quickly around the building and the next thing I knew was that I was standing on a chair in the middle of Court One displaying the knickers with the little swastikas. That morning there was an agent prosecutor who had never been to Epsom Magistrates' Court before. He did not know what planet he had landed on and we never saw him again. If such a thing happened today, I suspect that everyone involved would be put on a disciplinary charge, but this was all part of the *Life on Mars* workplace experience back in the day!

One of the questions I and my fellow defence lawyers are often asked revolves round how it is possible to act for clients who profess their innocence when the evidence presented points to their "obvious guilt". In other words, how can I act for someone I know to be guilty.

The answer is quite straightforward. It is not for me or any defence lawyer to decide on guilt – that is for the court. My role is to advise my client on evidence and plea. Yes, the evidence may be overwhelming and, yes, the advice may be to plead guilty. But as mentioned earlier if, at the end of the day, the client is adamant about their innocence, my role then is to put their case to court. I cannot knowingly allow a client to lie to the court but my opinion as to the truth is just that – opinion. I have always described myself as a glorified mouthpiece, putting a case to court in legalese that individuals may themselves not be able to do.

It is vital that our justice system allows individuals the opportunity to be heard fairly and reminds me of one of the first tenets taught at the outset of my law degree – it is better that ten guilty men go free than for one innocent man to be convicted.

Which leads me on to another question I am asked, although less frequently, namely, have I encountered any miscarriages of justice during my long career. Sadly, I have but they have been few in number and the circumstances have been such that the wrongs have eventually been righted and the impact on those affected has been mercifully light.

There is, however, one major exception that has had a devastating effect on the lives of innocent people wrongly accused and where the long-drawn-out remedial process remains in train over twenty years later. I am referring to the prosecution by the Post Office of large numbers of decent, honest and innocent sub-postmasters and mistresses across the country for theft and/or false accounting.

It was alleged by the Post Office that negative discrepancies in the accounts of the sub-post offices involved must be due to the misappropriation of the sums in question by the relevant sub-postmaster or mistress.

I was instructed to act on behalf of a number of the accused at the time and was immediately struck by the odd coincidence that so many pillars of the community, with no previous criminal records, had supposedly turned to fraud and dishonesty once taking on the running of a sub-post office.

There were suspicions about the robustness of the Post Office's accounting system but the organisation strongly resisted all suggestions of possible technical issues and denied proper access to defence forensic experts. It embarked on a strategy of misinformation and cover-up as it continued to prosecute each sub-postmaster or mistress with accounting losses, many of whom were told by the prosecutors that their "misdeeds" were unique. A majority of those so accused had plunged deep into debt through borrowing and remortgaging to make good the apparent losses. Many went to prison.

The corporate mendacity of the Post Office, and outrageous mistreatment of its sub-postmasters and mistresses, was only exposed through the campaigning resolve and persistence of those wrongly prosecuted, the support of their family, friends and communities, the involvement of a few proactive politicians and the tenacity of investigative journalists such as the award-winning Nick Wallis.

Gradually the Post Office IT system and inherent dishonesty were revealed as the true culprits, and subsequent court judgments have been damning. Nevertheless, the Post Office showed little remorse and the process of restitution through the courts continues. Meanwhile the sense of hurt and injustice remains, while some of those directly affected, sadly, have not lived to see the final outcome.

It is clearly not possible to do full justice to this distressing case here but more information can be found by listening to *The Great Post Office Trial* on BBC Sounds (and following related coverage on other current affairs programmes such as *Panorama* and *Inside Out*).

I have obviously been able to do no more here than scratch the surface of the types of case I have dealt with over the years. It is perhaps a cliché to say that no two cases have been alike. But it is the variety, coupled with the privilege of being able to advise and represent, to the very best of one's ability, vulnerable people at the most challenging times of their lives, that has made my career so rewarding and satisfying.

8

Soldiering On

There has never been a dull moment while operating within the civilian jurisdiction, but the military courts and their enforcement agencies have nevertheless done their utmost to ensure that they offer an even more colourful experience in comparison!

The UK military is subject to its own criminal justice system, with laws and processes that, in the majority of respects, closely mirror those that apply to the civilian population. It does, however, have its own investigative capability (performed by the Royal Military Police), prosecution arm (the Service Prosecution Authority) and court structure (Courts-Martial). The latter differ significantly from civilian courts in that they are presided over by a specialist military judge, known as a Judge Advocate, while decisions about guilt and innocence are determined by a board of – usually – between three and seven serving personnel rather than a jury consisting of twelve members of the public.

This separate system of justice is occasionally accused of being anachronistic and deficient by legal observers and the media, particularly after high-profile cases that are perceived to have led to perverse outcomes. Robert Sherrill wrote a book following a controversial court martial in the USA in the early Seventies and summed up his feelings by giving it the title *Military Justice is to Justice as Military Music is to Music*. But the military system survives as a separate entity, with a degree of consistency being offered by the fact that appeals from both civilian Crown Courts and military courts-martial are heard by the same cadre of appeal court judges.

Given the relatively small number of military personnel as a proportion of the general population, it is not common for defence lawyers to specialise in military as well as civilian law. It is, to some extent, regarded as a bit of a niche area of criminal law practice and those defence lawyers who decide to focus on military law either do so as a conscious decision based on experience or interest (e.g. because they trained as lawyers within a military setting) or because their office is located close to a large military camp or centre of population. I fall into the latter category, having spent a significant part of my career working in and around Aldershot with its strong military links and traditions.

As a result of building experience, expertise and a reputation within military circles, aided by the extent and frequency with which contacts in the military family move units and locations, it was not long before military cases represented around forty per cent of my total workload. This percentage has been sustained throughout my career and involved me in frequent business trips to British bases across the UK and Germany, as well as stays in Cyprus, Kenya, Brunei and the United States.

Every so often a military case will be dealt with by the civilian authorities, depending on the circumstances, and decisions taken by the respective investigative and prosecuting personnel. A most unusual case in this category occurred in 1997 when I was called out as duty solicitor to Guildford Police Station to represent Milos Stankovic who had been arrested by

Ministry of Defence (MOD) police for an alleged breach of the Official Secrets Act. I can name him because he subsequently wrote a book about his experiences.

He was a British Army officer with the UN peacekeeping force during the Bosnian War and acted as a high-level liaison officer between UN commanders and the likes of Radovan Karadžić and Slobodan Milošević. It was this that led to his arrest. Eventually, after two investigations and a High Court action, he was cleared. I only acted for him for a few months at the beginning of his ordeal because he clearly needed a specialist to take on the MOD in civil proceedings and that was outside my criminal law expertise. But, as a thank-you for my small part, he arranged for me to have lunch in the House of Commons with Martin Bell, the former MP who had campaigned vigorously on his behalf, and General Sir Michael Rose, commander of the UN forces during the war. I can still see myself relaxing on the Palace of Westminster balcony overlooking the Thames, sipping my second, hefty pre-lunch vodka and tonic. I also received a namecheck in Milos's book, *Trusted Mole*, and its serialisation in one of the Sunday broadsheets.

Because life in the military world is, of necessity, full of precise rules, rituals and practices, it can make for an amusing interlude when things sometimes go wrong. One such incident early in my career occurred at a trial at the court-martial centre in Aldershot. At that time courts-martial were pompous, stuffy affairs and, yes, there was lots of marching, lots of it . . .

The courtroom was a long thin room with only one door to enter by. The prosecution and defence tables faced each other along the side walls. Across the end was the bench where the Judge Advocate would join the Army Board members to preside over this heinous case.

In due course my client, the accused, would be sitting in front of my table facing the bench, leaving just enough room for the Judge Advocate to pass through and join the board before proceedings could commence.

So, we were set to go.

The prosecutor, Colonel Straitjacket, was standing rigidly to attention behind his table, fixing me with a disapproving stare, clearly believing my civilian attempt to do attention was shambolic.

Members of the board – Brigadier Bigot, Colonel Cocksure and Major Misanthrope – had scrubbed up well in their No 2 uniforms dripping in shiny leather, braid and medals.

Court Orderly Foghorn bellowed, "The court is now *open*!! March in the accused!! Left!! Left!! Left!!"

Judge Advocate Bluster followed, gown flowing behind him. It was his first day, first case. As he passed through between the prosecution and defence tables, he knocked over the prosecution water jug. Water went everywhere but there was not the minutest of flickers from Colonel Straitjacket.

"Ah," Bluster flapped. "I'll withdraw while this is cleared up."

"The court is now *closed*!! March out the accused!! Left!! Left!! Left!!" bellowed Court Orderly Foghorn again.

The mess was cleared up.

"The court is now *open*!! March in the accused!! Left!! Left!! Left!!" was roared out yet again by Foghorn.

There was still no flicker from Colonel Straitjacket as Judge Advocate Bluster made it successfully to the bench. By now my sides were beginning to split!

My client, Private Pitiful, was a lowly clerk, lacking any obvious star quality. His odious crime was to have stolen a load of travel warrants, which he made out to Penzance or John O'Groats then sold to his mates, who readily bought them even though none had ever lived in, or been to, either of these places.

So it fell to Judge Advocate Bluster to read out the charges to Private Pitiful. He droned on in a monotonous tone. *On such and such a day you made out a travel warrant from Aldershot to Penzance. On such and such a day you made out a travel warrant from Aldershot to John O'Groats* and on and on and on.

Finally, he got to the twentieth and last charge. *On such and such a day you made out a travel warrant from AlderSHIT to—*

The balloon of pomposity totally burst. I completely lost it and nearly ended up on my own charge of contempt of court! But I was full of silent admiration for my military friends and adversaries who, unlike me, had clearly been trained not to corpse, as they say in theatrical circles, in the face of adversity.

Moving seamlessly from stolen travel warrants to alleged war crimes, I was instructed in 2006 to represent a staff sergeant who was accused, alongside six others, of beating to death a suspected insurgent, Baha Mousa, while in British Army custody in Iraq in 2003. It was a most interesting case with the trial itself, which took place at Bulford Military Court Centre in Wiltshire, lasting over six months. It was later the subject of a public inquiry, which published its report in 2011.

The court staff provided each of the seven defence teams with a dedicated office for the duration of the trial at Bulford. This was extremely helpful because it meant we could set up a storage facility for our hundreds of ring binders of evidence rather than take them with us each day. I made a number of trips to the local stationer for our copious requirements, including a small printer. We also bought other indispensable items of equipment such as a coffee-making machine and a kettle.

Our room was immediately opposite the one that was turned into the temporary scoff house (to borrow a military phrase) so we were able to have first dibs on the daily lunches provided by the catering corps. Such service – you would not get that in a civilian court.

Most of the time I travelled to and from Bulford every day – a journey of no more than fifty minutes each way. During school holidays there were some days when I had no option but to take Leah, then aged nine, with me. She still remembers sitting in our room with her books and Nintendo DS. Later, when aged fifteen, she enjoyed doing some work experience in the Bulford court office.

Occasionally, when we were working late or starting early, my QC insisted that I stay over, which I did at the Red Lion in Salisbury. During one of those stays he had a special dinner commitment at the Bleeding Heart restaurant in central London, to which I was invited. It was a very enjoyable dinner, finishing in the early hours. I barely had anything to drink because I was so tired and was worried about falling asleep at the table. I was looking forward to sleeping in the taxi on the way back to Salisbury, but it was not to be.

It was one of those interesting experiences when you find yourself the only truly sober member of a rather convivial assembly. The noise made by the others in the taxi was unbelievable until they all fell asleep. By then I was wide awake with sleep a distant prospect.

We got back to the Red Lion at 4 a.m. The maid had left the window open and my room was freezing cold. At 6 a.m. my phone rang – my sharp and fully functioning QC wanted to start work. How did he, and others like him, do it?

During the trial it was planned that the court would go on a site visit to Basra in Iraq. What an unusual opportunity for a civilian. The intention was to be based at the international airport and be flown by Chinook helicopter into the city centre where all the action germane to the trial had taken place.

I had had all my jabs in preparation, my bergen was packed and we had received our movement orders from RAF Brize Norton. Unfortunately, due to a sudden deterioration in the security situation, the trip was cancelled at the last minute and was not rescheduled. What a disappointment, although I think that there were many in my family who did not agree with that sentiment! Funnily enough, Basra never reappeared on my bucket list – business or social!

To cut a long story – or trial – short, my client was acquitted, along with those others who had pleaded not guilty. Given the outcome, and enormous cost to the public purse of both trial and inquiry, I am sure even then that ministers would have said, as they always do, that lessons will be learned. But as we all know, they rarely are!

Another court martial linked to Op Telic, the name given to operations covering the presence of our troops in Iraq both during and after the war, took place at Catterick Military Court Centre in 2007. I represented a soldier accused of running guns and ammunition into Germany from Iraq. He was one of three defendants alleged to have been involved in this nefarious practice during his tour on Op Telic. My client was acquitted after a trial lasting two months. For the duration of the trial our team, consisting of two barristers, the defending officer (an officer routinely assigned by the military to assist personnel facing disciplinary or criminal charges) and myself, stayed, on Vinny's recommendation, at The Buck Inn in the charming village of Thornton Watlass, about fifteen minutes' drive from Catterick Garrison. Why, you might ask, was Vinny in a position to recommend a village pub in North Yorkshire? Well, that's a story in itself, which I think is worth sharing.

In the Nineties Vinny was summonsed to give evidence at an employment tribunal in Leeds involving an Immigration Service employee claiming unfair dismissal. The tribunal was set to last a week and the regional manager, who reported to Vinny, was also due to give evidence. They stayed in a nondescript hotel in central Leeds and after the regional manager had completed his evidence on the Tuesday, he suggested that they travel the forty-seven miles to his home in Thornton Watlass for a more relaxing evening, including a meal in The Buck Inn. The regional manager would drive both ways and ensure that Vinny was back for his evidence session starting at 10 a.m. the following morning. Vinny bought into the plan, albeit rather reluctantly.

The two of them did indeed spend a very pleasant and relaxing evening at The Buck Inn and enjoyed a good night's sleep. Unfortunately, and contrary to the weather forecast, it snowed heavily overnight and the two of them woke early the following morning to find the village cut off.

Luckily, the regional manager was friends with the local farmer, who came to the rescue by driving them in his powerful tractor to Northallerton Railway Station from where the odd train was running. While hanging on to the tractor as it made its hazardous twenty-one-mile journey across the snowbound and deserted North Yorkshire countryside, Vinny was attempting to construct an explanation as to why he might be arriving late at the tribunal when based just a few doors away in the centre of Leeds.

Through sheer good luck the tractor's arrival at Northallerton Station coincided with a train bound for Leeds that, although running slowly, got them to the tribunal with two minutes to spare. Vinny walked nonchalantly in and gave his evidence as though nothing untoward had happened that morning . . . and the employee lost his claim.

Returning to my dastardly story, I have to say The Buck Inn was a perfect base. There were only eight bedrooms of which we had four so, for the majority of the time, we were the only residents. The pub had a lovely garden and, given the wonderful September weather prevailing at the time, we were able to sit out in the afternoons after court, surrounded by case papers and laptops, preparing for the following day. My client was also able to join us for conferences.

The evenings cooled quickly so dinner was taken in the bar with a fire roaring in the grate. The locals would come in and enjoy drinks with the strange bunch of southerners who had temporarily taken over the pub.

All in all, if one had to be away for a lengthy trial, this was surely one of the better ways of surviving. It became home from home and we more or less had the run of the place.

If I could get away for the weekend, I would do so, which meant flying between Teesside and Heathrow. I loved those flights because the weather was invariably good and flying down the east side of the country made me appreciate just how rural much of England is.

One Monday morning I got the red-eye back up to Teesside, arriving at the pub in time for breakfast. I let myself in through the back door of the kitchen and made a very noisy and grandiose entrance into the bar where breakfast was set up. The rest of the team greeted me equally exuberantly.

At this point I was vaguely aware of another table being occupied by, so I thought, an unknown couple. The team went off to gather their gubbins for the day ahead, leaving me to enjoy a cup of coffee in the now silent bar. Then a voice chirped up from said other table. "Morning, Issy!" I turned. It was only a friend and former colleague of Vinny's, together with his wife, enjoying a few days away from their home in Devon. And I had just made a complete spectacle of myself!

Many of the courts-martial that I defended in took place in the Military Court Centre in Sennelager, near Paderborn, Germany, where until recently there was a significant British military presence. However, I also visited further-flung British Army outposts on a less frequent basis. The British Army garrison in Brunei, which is largely funded by the sultan, counts among that number. I was asked to act for a client there when the original RAF lawyer declared a conflict with himself in the police interview. I never quite understood how he managed to do that!

The first trip was hurriedly put together at the last minute. I flew to Singapore with Qantas. That was an experience in itself. It was the 2 January 2012. The cabin crew were incredibly rude. The plane was full of Aussie families returning after Christmas. As soon as one crying baby fell asleep, another started. I arrived in Singapore, with eyes propped open by matchsticks, to await a connecting Royal Brunei flight to Bandar Seri Begawan (a cracking capital-cities answer on BBC's *Pointless*!).

As a Muslim country Brunei is supposedly alcohol-free. I was aware that foreign nationals visiting the country are allowed to take in alcohol for personal use. Consequently, while waiting at Singapore Changi Airport I purchased a half bottle of whisky, purely of course for medicinal purposes. I completed the requisite form and duly declared said bottle on arrival at BSB, only to be asked by the customs official whether I was sure I had brought enough alcohol with me!

I stayed a few nights on that, and a subsequent occasion, in the officers' mess in the British Forces Brunei garrison at Seria. A charming colonial residence from which I could walk straight on to the beach overlooking the South China Sea.

Returning home through Singapore, as a present from Vinny, I spent the night at Raffles Hotel – another wonderfully colonial experience.

Vinny also bought me a guidebook on the top twenty-five Singaporean sights. I left the hotel at around 8 a.m. the following morning and took a taxi out to the botanical gardens. Delightful. I wended my way back on foot, returning to Raffles about 8 p.m. having ticked off eleven of the twenty-five sights.

After a Singapore Sling or three at the top of the neighbouring Stamford Tower taking in the night views, I headed to the airport for the midnight flight home.

Later that year a third visit saw me back in Brunei, this time for the trial. The whole flight was on Royal Brunei but via Dubai instead. Vinny has not forgotten receiving a middle-of-the-night call from Barclaycard, querying why our card was in use in Dubai. He had to explain (while trembling, I am sure, at the thought of the forthcoming bill) that I must be in the duty-free shop at Dubai Airport!

For logistical reasons the defence team stayed this time at a hotel in Kuala Belait, near to Seria. Although we had been made honorary members of the NAAFI to assist us with our needs, we did avail ourselves of some excellent local restaurants. Again, alcohol was off the menu but it was amazing what came out of the teapots provided with the meals!

The trial itself presented a number of unique and interesting challenges, including some that revolved around cultural differences and interpretation. It demonstrated, yet again, the diversity and distinctive nature of court-martial casework.

Another court martial that presented new and tricky challenges with a strong international flavour took place in the years 2016 and 2017. The charge faced by my client arose out of an incident that took place at a United Nations (UN) military conference in Kampala, Uganda. There were a number of potential witnesses based in Kenya and Somalia who needed to be interviewed as part of the trial preparation. I therefore flew to Nairobi for a week where I was able to take a number of defence witness statements.

Additionally, I was due to travel from Nairobi to Mogadishu for further statement-gathering but unfortunately the security logistics were deemed to be too problematic when the appointed time arrived.

The majority of prosecution witnesses were American citizens. It was therefore decided that the prosecution case should be held at Andrews Airforce Base in Maryland, just outside Washington DC, with the defence case following at Bulford Military Court Centre back in the UK.

The "best" hotel the defence team could find close to the Andrews Airforce Base was the Holiday Inn Express at Camp Springs, and staying there proved an interesting experience to say the least. We were able to take over the small business centre as a work area because there were few business customers in the hotel. Unfortunately, the reason for the lack of business customers was the presence of noisy children in swarm-like numbers, all on regulation school trips to Washington DC. The irony was that when I commented that the bill was higher than originally quoted on *Booking.com*, I was told it was because of "full occupancy". My complaint, that full occupancy was only due to legions of rowdy schoolchildren who had disrupted our stay, fell on deaf ears.

The hotel's facilities were nondescript and the restaurants in the immediate vicinity left a lot to be desired. It did, however, mean that we had to take Ubers down to the National Harbor area on the Potomac River in downtown Washington DC, which more than made up for the deprivations suffered at the hands of the Holiday Inn Express.

For the purposes of the prosecution case, a courtroom in the airbase was designated as a British military court. We had a vehicle at our disposal to transport the defence team between the hotel and base. If we did not make it out of the base by 5 p.m. each evening we had to stand still wherever we were, along with everyone else, while the American national anthem was played.

By the time the trial commenced, one of the prosecution witnesses had been posted to Islamabad. It did seem somewhat surreal sitting in an American airbase, in a room designated as British soil, listening to video evidence from Pakistan.

The major problem in preparing the defence case was having to deal with the UN. While the organisation indicated, on the face of it, its willingness to assist, we had to follow strict protocol and the expression *time is of the essence* clearly did not feature in its lexicon. My client was adamant that a UN laptop, used in Kampala by the main prosecution witness, would contain supportive evidence critical to his defence. Naturally we wanted it examined by our forensic expert. But the laptop was, by then, back in the UN HQ in New York with the UN refusing to allow it to be shipped to the UK for the purposes of the trial.

The trial had already been adjourned once due to the delays caused by the UN's convoluted ways of working and, not surprisingly, the Judge Advocate General would not countenance another. Unnervingly, we found ourselves in a situation where our forensic expert, accompanied by that of the prosecution from the Special Investigation Branch (SIB) of the Royal Military Police, had to fly to New York to examine the laptop just as the trial was commencing in Washington.

When the defence case commenced back in the UK, our forensic expert was still in New York with the SIB officer. Finally, at the eleventh hour, the expert's report arrived. As anticipated, it contained vital evidence that played a significant part in my client being acquitted. Talk about a close shave, Gromit!

It is highly improbable that such complicated logistics would be contemplated in the current environment, and I suspect that the necessary evidence-gathering and trial process would in future rely more heavily on modern technology. Whether or not that will result in swifter and better justice remains to be seen.

In another high-profile court-martial case, with links to terrorism and potential reprisals, I was provided with Special Branch protection in my role as one of the defence lawyers. The nature of the protection mainly consisted of a liaison officer being assigned to me and my close family, and our house and vehicles being kept under remote surveillance.

Late one night during the course of the court martial there was a knock at our front door. I had just gone to bed so it fell to Vinny to answer. Much to my consternation, given the late hour, I heard the caller being invited in. In my semi-conscious state, I was convinced that the voice I could hear was that of a perpetually drunken and troublesome local client whom I was keen to avoid. In a bizarre attempt to extricate Vinny from what I mistakenly believed to be a tricky situation, I dragged Leah out of bed and told her to go downstairs and request her father's assistance in removing a mouse from her room.

A few minutes later a very embarrassed and disgruntled Leah returned. I had to get out of bed and go down because the person Vinny had invited in was not a drunken client but a Special Branch officer. It transpired that our address had been picked up from an online chat that they were monitoring so wanted to provide some further security advice. I never did ask the officer whether he was any good at phantom mouse-catching!

It was just as well that we informed our immediate neighbours of the remote surveillance because, on another occasion, they found armed response officers peering over their fence after our burglar alarm had malfunctioned. It was reassuring to know that our interests were being so well looked after, but I think our neighbours were relieved when the trial was over and they could return to tending their vegetable patch without being rudely interrupted by gun-toting police.

As with my career providing advice and support to clients in a civilian setting, I have drawn enormous intellectual stimulation and satisfaction from representing service personnel accused of a wide range of criminal offences while on or off duty. Moreover, I have been privileged to have met, and worked with or against, so many gifted professionals whose sole objective has been to ensure that justice is done – and done fairly – in both areas of the criminal law. I feel fortunate indeed to reflect that so many of my fellow professionals will remain firm and lifelong friends.

9

Vinny and Leah

It will come as no surprise to you that the two most important people in my life are my husband, Vinny, and my daughter, Leah.

I first met Vinny in July 1983. It was at a wedding in Shenfield, Essex. At the time my late first husband, Julian, and Vinny worked together in what was then HM Customs and Excise (now part of Her Majesty's Revenue and Customs). They were VAT inspectors based in Soho, central London, which as you can imagine produced some entertaining experiences. One of their colleagues was getting married and consequently a venue of VAT officers (fittingly also the collective noun for vultures) was present.

I have to admit that I found the reception extremely tedious, not helped by the fact that I became trapped in a corner by a dry nerd explaining the ins and outs of a certain VAT form known as a 000CV – pronounced *triple nought CV* . . . I have never forgotten it!

Thankfully, I was not the only one suffering from boredom. It was not long before Julian, myself, Vinny and his then wife, Gwen, extricated ourselves and decamped to a local Italian restaurant.

That marked the start of a long-standing friendship. Throughout the Eighties we socialised on a regular basis. As Julian and I lived in Hampshire, while Vinny and Gwen lived in Kent, the social events usually took the form of dinner at our respective houses, trips to the theatre or, naturally, visits to live sports events. But it was not unusual for Vinny and Julian to head off to the cricket and for Gwen and me to find alternative entertainment, despite my love of cricket – e.g. a Bruce Springsteen concert at Wembley during his 1984 *Born in the USA* tour!

In 1989 Vinny and Gwen drifted apart. Gwen's career took her to Manchester while Vinny was based close to his office in Croydon, Surrey. By this time Vinny had moved from HM Customs and Excise via the Passport Office to become an assistant chief inspector in the Immigration Service (now the UK Border Force). Although we remained in contact during the Nineties, we saw less of him socially as his busy Home Office career increasingly consumed more of his time and necessitated frequent periods away on domestic and international business.

In 1999 Julian suddenly died of hypertrophic cardio-myopathy. It came as a total shock as we were unaware that he was suffering from any illness. He was forty-one, I was thirty-nine and Leah was just two years old at the time.

I had not seen Vinny since 1997 when he, Julian and I had attended a Test Match together at The Oval. Naturally, I made contact to let Vinny know of Julian's unexpected death. Thereafter we saw each other socially and our friendship quickly developed in a direction that neither of us would previously have anticipated. We married in 2000, and in 2001 he adopted Leah. The process meant that, rather bizarrely, I also had to adopt her at the same time!

We were married on the enormous balcony of our room at Le Victoria Hotel in the district of Pamplemousse on the island of Mauritius. Leah was our bridesmaid/flower girl and our witnesses were the guest liaison officer and the head waiter. A superbly simple affair.

As it was a special holiday, we travelled in business class. It gave Leah a taste for comfort that has remained with her! We stayed for three weeks. During that time Leah was the star of the show, mastering water skiing aged just three, making the most of Mini Club and generally enjoying the dining opportunities.

As an aside, while there we also earned brownie points with my cricket-loving mother. We had tickets for the Lord's Test against the West Indies, which we passed to my mother, who took one of her oldest friends. It was the second day and quite extraordinary. The West Indies' first innings closed with the first ball of the day. England then succumbed abjectly to being all out for 134. However, they turned the tables on the Windies and bowled them out for 54 before batting again – and going on to win the game the following day!

It meant that my mother witnessed all or part of four Test innings in a single day, a rare occurrence indeed. We actually felt quite envious relaxing on a sunny beach thousands of miles away!

A few days after our return from Mauritius, I received a fax from someone in the court administration office. It was addressed to Mrs Hagg. When responding I corrected the spelling to *Hogg* and pointed out that I was now a pig, not a witch (although technically a *hogg* with two g's, is a sheep)!

It was our twentieth wedding anniversary in June 2020 but Covid-19 restrictions put paid to our intended celebrations. We should have been off to Twickers to enjoy watching the

Gallagher Premiership Rugby Final, not that we purchased the tickets many months previously in the hope or expectation that our team, Bath Rugby, might be there. It just happens to be an excellent day out.

Instead, our anniversary commenced with Claire Balding's *Ramblings* on Radio 4 – another coincidence in that it was a compilation marking twenty years since the programme started. We also watched the New Zealand rugby match between Chiefs and Blues to make up for the loss of live fare at Twickenham.

On informing Vinny that a twentieth anniversary was marked with china, he responded by noting the irony (and harmony) given the prevailing circumstances, but still did not fancy celebrating with an imported case of coronavirus from Wuhan.

Vinny continued his career in the Home Office until he retired in 2011 after forty-two years as a civil servant. I think it quite remarkable that having been brought up in care by the Children's Society following the death of his mother when he was aged five, then the subsequent abandonment by his father a year or so later, and leaving school at the age of sixteen, he still managed to progress to fill a number of important senior positions within one of the great departments of state. In 2009 he was made a Companion of the Order of the Bath in the Queen's Birthday Honours. But Vinny is a modest, self-effacing individual who simply counts himself lucky to have had the opportunity to play his small part in an important area of public life.

Not content to don his slippers or golf shoes on retiring, while I continued on my unremitting tour of police stations, courts and courts martial, Vinny embarked on a second, consultancy career. This saw him engage with the likes of EY (formerly known as Ernst and Young) in Paris and DCAF in Geneva on a range of projects as far afield as Stockholm, Dublin, Vienna, The Hague, Yerevan and Tbilisi.

Towards the latter part of his civil service career, the need to commute to London from north-east Hampshire, combined with the nature of his work, made for very long days, catching the 6.35 a.m. train from Winchfield and rarely returning home before 8 p.m. But such journeys were not without the odd flash of humour.

There was a late-night episode several years ago when two regular commuters were sitting opposite each other. In a typically British way they obviously knew each other and their regular habits, but such familiarity did not extend to the art of conversation. One of the commuters, Mr Rude, was resting his head against the window in a partial drunken slumber. As the train approached Fleet his fellow traveller, Mr Anxious, kept leaning across looking for signs of consciousness. Eventually, Mr Anxious felt he needed to take decisive action as follows.

> *Mr Anxious: (roughly shaking Mr Rude awake) "I'm sorry, sir, but I have seen you get off here many times. I thought you should know we are coming into Fleet."*
>
> *Mr Rude: (groggily coming to, wiping condensation off the window and peering out) "Why don't you **** off. I've moved."*

On another occasion, Vinny was travelling with a delightful, larger-than-life character who, sadly, is no longer with us. For the sake of argument, I shall call said character Gus (which is handy because that was also his real name).

Sitting opposite each other on the adjoining table were two nuns who suddenly became bothered by a wasp. Gus, donning his virtual Good Samaritan armour, rolled up his newspaper, stretched across between the two nuns and, with a loud thud, splatted the errant wasp against the train window. The two nuns simultaneously screamed at both the action and resultant mess, to which Gus simply said, "Don't worry, my dears, he's in the bosom of Abraham now!!"

Such gallantry and panache!

Gus's ability to inadvertently shock those in esteemed positions with words or deeds was once matched by someone closer to home. When Leah was three, Vinny took her to Toys R Us, very much expecting her to choose yet another cuddly giraffe, tiger or rat. Much to his surprise, she bypassed the soft toy department and made a beeline for the dolls, selecting a smartly dressed young lady whom she subsequently called Amy. Vinny was delighted that Leah demonstrated her fully ingrained egalitarian principles at such an early age by choosing the only black doll in the shop.

Like many three-year old children, Leah was at the stage when she was beginning to pick up the odd word or phrase subliminally and storing them without necessarily understanding the true meaning or context.

Not surprisingly, one day Leah took Amy to nursery with her. She was met at the door by the manageress, Mrs Po-face, who started the following conversation.

Mrs Po-face: "Hello, Leah. What a lovely doll. Is she new?"

Leah: "Yes. Daddy gave her to me."

Mrs Po-face: "Does she have a name?"

Leah: "Amy and it's her birthday today."

Mrs Po-face "And what does Amy want for her birthday?"

Leah: "Political asylum!"

There was much sucking-in of teeth by Mrs Po-face. I had to draw on my finely tuned advocacy skills to convince the teacher that we had not been schooling our daughter in far right propaganda to avoid being drummed out of nursery.

I am pleased to say that Mrs Po-face quickly identified the innocence of extreme youth and we were soon back to being *personae gratae* at the nursery. It had a good reputation and offered children a wide range of learning activities and events.

One Easter it set the children the task of painting a hard-boiled egg in attractive patterns and colours and then taking it, or sending it, on a journey that they then had to narrate. Leah mentioned this task to Vinny one weekend, who offered to take the egg into Number 10 Downing Street as part of its adventure. (He thought it inappropriate to use the word "smuggle", which this part of the egg's journey would entail.)

Leah readily agreed to the plan, so Vinny took the egg into Number 10 the following week, slightly concerned as to what he might say if the sensors at the security gates leading into Downing Street identified either the shape or smell of the egg. Given his role at the time – namely Director of Drugs Strategy – arguing that the contraband must have been planted would not have sounded plausible!

Fortuitously, he managed to proceed through security, and so later sat opposite the PM in the cabinet room at Number 10, engaged, no doubt, in debate about weighty matters of state with Leah's painted egg safely nestled in his suit pocket. Leah naturally included this element of her egg's sojourn in her overall travelogue that, I seem to recall, was both varied and inventive.

Back at the nursery Mrs Po-face was less than amused. She gave the impression that Leah must have let her imagination run far too wild. So much for encouraging creativity!

Vinny never liked to bring his work persona home with him, preferring to leave it very much at the office door. But there were the odd occasions when he felt the need to take charge of a situation. Consequently, Vinny *having a word* has become a bit of a family catchphrase. Leah and I know that when he says this in response to any situation, it is best for us to melt into the shadows and leave him to it.

Many years ago, on our way to a half-term cottage holiday in Cornwall, we stayed the night in a very smart hotel on Bodmin Moor. Our charming room was more than ample for the three of us. But we had to call housekeeping as soon as we arrived. There was insufficient bedding and a lack of tea-making facilities. To cap it all, in the morning there was no hot water.

As we were about to check out, Vinny said, "I think I'll have a word with the manager." Time for me to take Leah to the car and wait. Vinny joined us shortly thereafter – fifty per cent off the bill!

I recall another occasion when I worked in Basingstoke and my office was located opposite a local homeless shelter. One day I discovered that my car had been keyed all down one side (despite the fact that, as a firm, we represented a number of residents when they stepped over the legal line). Vinny visited the shelter and had a quiet word. My car was never touched again.

A similar incident requiring *a word* occurred one Saturday when we had planned to go to London. The train line between Basingstoke and Woking was closed due to engineering works. Our only option was to drive to Guildford and catch the train from there. At the time Vinny had an annual season ticket, which as many will know, represents a serious financial investment. At Guildford ticket office Vinny produced his season ticket and explained that our line was closed. The ticket operative wanted to charge Vinny £2.16, the fare from Guildford to Brookwood being that small part of the journey not covered by the annual season ticket. Vinny had a word. He did not have to pay.

In 2011 an academic and former BBC home affairs correspondent gave Vinny a book he had just published entitled, *Crime, Policy and the Media: The Shaping of Criminal Justice*. He did so because he had cited an issue in which Vinny had been involved. I will not bore you with the context but the pertinent passage read, "*. . . this caused some alarm amongst ministers and . . . Vic Hogg almost certainly 'had words' with . . . [the protagonist]*".

Vinny's occasionally unconventional approach once led him to decline an invitation to a Royal Garden Party because it clashed with a Test Match at Lord's. However, he did not blot his copybook as, to my slight envy, he was invited to have lunch with the Queen and Duke of Edinburgh at Buckingham Palace in 2006, alongside seven other invitees from diverse walks of life. Including members of the Royal Household, there were only twelve attendees for a three-hour lunch – excluding the corgis of course. Vinny met one of the other invitees, a well-known travel writer, in the loos prior to the proceedings. They had to admit to each other that the "urge to go" was generated by idle curiosity more than any utilitarian need.

Given the Queen's interest in all things military, Vinny managed to weave into the conversation a high-profile court martial that I was involved with at the time. Not only was the Queen conversant with all the *dramatis personae*, but she knew the precise nature of the background and issues as well as the stage of the proceedings! Very impressive.

I did at least get to see the Queen at Vinny's investiture as a Companion of the Order of the Bath in 2009 (Leah and I had second row seats) and again at a Westminster Abbey service for members of the Order in 2014 when Vinny earned brownie points by also inviting my mother to attend.

It is typical of Vinny that he rarely mentions these and other experiences and plays them down when raised. Following the lunch, I gathered together the invitation, menu, seating plan, name place, court circular and so on to form a montage that hangs in a hidden corner of our dining room. If you asked Vinny his favourite Queen story, he would probably say the time when Gerry Queen, the former Crystal Palace player, was sent off at Selhurst Park in the early Seventies for fighting in a game against Arsenal. One newspaper's headline the following day ran *Queen in Brawl at Palace!*

I have already touched on a couple of incidents from Leah's time at nursery school which, I am sure, helped to encourage the independent spirit that she demonstrated at a very early age. She was never afraid to say or do her own thing, as demonstrated by the story above about her doll named Amy. On a later occasion one of the nursery teachers was very pleased to inform me that Leah, at such a young age, had shown very good concentration by watching a video for five minutes without being distracted. I had to disappoint the teacher by pointing out that Leah was hoodwinking her because she was more than capable of concentrating for at least half an hour.

This concentration was put to dubious use when Leah and a couple of young friends decided to free the guinea pigs from their hutch, a foretaste of Leah's prosocial and humanitarian leanings.

While Leah was still at nursery, I took her for an interview at The Grey House, a preparatory school in Hartley Wintney, Hampshire. I remember with such clarity this introductory visit to the school. Leah must have been two, coming up for three. We started in the office of the redoubtable headmistress, Mrs Purse, where she talked about the school and then took us on a tour, including showing us a lesson in progress. As we entered Form 6 the whole class rose in absolute unison and chimed, "Good morning, Mrs Purse." It gave me goosebumps!

We returned to her office for further discussions and I soon realised that it was me that was being interviewed – would I meet her exacting standards? I can still hear her words ringing in my ears, spoken on learning that Leah's parents were a lawyer and a senior civil servant, "Ah good. We don't like new money here." I think I passed!

It was a perfect school for Leah, one class of about twenty pupils per year, traditional values but by no means old-fashioned, its motto *In minimus fidelis*. Leah has the fondest of memories of her time there. One of my oldest and dearest friends, Sue Cooper, was Leah's Form K (kindergarten) teacher. She had the measure of Leah and, in her end-of-term Form K year report, summed Leah up to a tee by observing that "in an ideal world Leah will set her own agenda".

As a very small child, like many, Leah was very much into dinosaurs and wanted to be a palaeontologist (she could even say the word). She soon moved on to live animals and has been an avid fan of Marwell Zoo in Hampshire from a very early age. While obviously not comfortable with the animals' restriction of movement in comparison to their natural habitat, she is an admirer of Marwell's conservation and breeding programmes. Consequently, visiting different zoos has often been a feature of our various breaks, both in the UK and far beyond.

One of Leah's favourites was Taronga Zoo in Sydney, wonderfully positioned overlooking the city and harbour. Quite a small establishment but animal welfare appears to be a high concern.

Since we visited in 2014 a second has opened in Sydney, imaginatively called Sydney Zoo, that appears to have adopted a safari park concept. Leah's reaction to the opening was to wonder at a beautiful city that could host two zoological gardens!

Some of these places are perhaps more inclined to major on being visitor attractions rather than conservation programmes and they do, therefore, create a modicum of discomfort. Schönbrun Zoo in Vienna was pleasant but small, ARTIS in

Amsterdam left a lot to be desired, while Berlin Zoo bordered on the bizarre.

In fairness we did visit the latter in 2003 when we took my mother to Berlin for a long weekend for her seventy-fifth birthday. Much may have changed since. We stayed at the Hotel Adlon overlooking the Brandenburg Gate, which is actually in the old East Berlin. It was very obvious that large sums of money had been spent on improving that side of the city since reunification. But as soon as we passed through the Brandenburg Gate into the old West Berlin, it seemed the area had been neglected and become jaded, including Tiergarten, the area where the zoo is situated.

While walking through the park to the zoo entrance we witnessed a number of interesting assignations. Although it was typical inner-city parkland, and broad daylight, the area was clearly a popular spot for ladies of the night. Syringes and other paraphernalia could be spotted at various points *en route*. A questionable scene to explain to a six-year-old girl and her seventy-five-year-old grandmother!

Stockholm Zoo provided a memorable visit with its vast colonies of ring-tailed lemurs enjoying a licence to roam, and we have always enjoyed our various visits to zoos and safari parks located closer to home, such as Regent's Park, Whipsnade, Longleat and Woburn.

Perhaps one of the most unexpected zoo incidents that I experienced took place about thirty years ago at Beijing Zoo. Those of a certain age will recall that, as small children, we would stretch the side of our eyes into slits when referring to Chinese people. Obviously not an acceptable practice today but I am talking about a generation ago. While walking through

Beijing Zoo, and being the only Westerners around, we were approached by a school group of giggling four- or five-year-old Chinese children. They stood in front of us and stretched their eyes wide from top to bottom to make them round!

As a family we have been lucky enough to have travelled a great deal and had some remarkable holidays. Following Leah's enjoyable experience in Mauritius, we thought mini clubs would remain a part of our summer holidays for a while. That was until we went to Sardinia when she was five years old. The hotel rooms were in single-storey terraces in the gardens alongside paths that splayed out from the main walkway running through the centre of the grounds. On our first full day we took Leah to Mini Club and returned to settle down on the patio outside our room to enjoy the sun and beautiful gardens. Ten minutes later we spied Leah, on her own, trotting down our path to join us. Her explanation was that she could not stay at Mini Club because they did not speak English. Naturally, we were appalled that she could just walk out. Consequently, she did not return.

Only very recently, when reminiscing about this, I expressed my surprise to Leah that she had found her way back to us so easily. She admitted that on the way to Mini Club, she had counted the paths in order to find her way back. She'd clearly had no intention of staying!

Because of this independent spirit, Vinny and I often resorted to silly rhymes in order to provoke a more co-operative approach . . . with mixed success. For example, on a trip to Reykjavik when she was only three, Leah appeared to assume that it was her role to clear all the snow off every park bench after visiting a frozen and inhospitable farmyard zoo. On gently remonstrating with her, she reacted with particular stubbornness so we recited the following.

"Horsey, horsey, don't you stop,
I've just met a Leah in a terrible strop.
Her eyes were running and her nose was too.
Take her back to the farmyard zoo!"

But we quickly cheered her up by taking her to Tjornin Lake in the city centre to feed the swans and geese.

In Morocco she walked everywhere so slowly that Vinny invented the following.

"Won't you walk a little faster said the turtle to the frog;
there's a human right behind us and I think it's Leah Hogg."

Leah's independent spirit has also brought some entertaining exchanges, such as when she fell over, aged four, on uneven ground in Cyprus. On our simultaneously reminding her that we had forewarned of this eventuality should she continue to run around recklessly, she simply got up, brushed herself down and said, "I wish you two would talk one at a time instead of two at a time!"

Some months later, in Ghent, she fell fully clothed into the hotel outdoor pool after running around the surrounding sloping edge. The other guests were horrified when we simply burst out laughing over our coffees. Little did they know that she would have no difficulty getting out of the pool, which she did like a character in a slapstick comedy.

The reason we knew that falling in the pool would cause her no difficulty was because of her excellent aptitude for swimming, again demonstrated early on; by the age of six she had attained her mile badge.

She continued this early promise through her time at Grey House and was captain of the swimming team that won the English Schools Swimming Association national relay championship, coming home with gold and silver medals. After local and regional rounds, we attended the nationals at the Ponds Forge International Sports Centre pool in Sheffield. The team was led by the sports teacher, inspirational former professional footballer Colin Smith, who encouraged them by urging, "You don't win silver, you lose gold!"

After "winning" silver in the medley, he made the reluctant team congratulate the gold medallists. The psychology worked and our team won gold in the freestyle, bringing home the national championship. Not bad for a school of only 150 pupils!

The train journey home was entertaining. The champagne flowed among the adults and our party was rather boisterous, but fellow passengers were very understanding and some even joined in. The guard announced the win over the tannoy and the winning team were allowed time in the driver's cab.

Next, we were joined by a former Grey House pupil who was returning with her father from a university open day and had heard the announcement. A small world!

Leah also swam competitively for Alton, but as time progressed it became clear that she and 5 a.m. training stints were not going to be natural bedfellows! When her interest began to wane, she profoundly said to me, "Whatever happens, they can't take my national medals away." Too right, Leah!

For a short while, alongside swimming, Leah developed an interest in horse riding as do many young girls of that age. It was fairly short-lived and came to an end when she was thrown from her horse during a hack. It reminded me of my own similar experience when my interest in riding was ended by a Shetland pony called Kingpin throwing me then biting me in the back.

In addition to swimming, netball and horse riding, Leah also tried her hand at cricket with Fleet Cricket Club, being selected for Hampshire North as a wicketkeeper/batsman. She also won bronze at a one-off judo competition.

Once past the competitive sporting phases, Leah became a bit of a petrol head. She was a huge fan of *Top Gear*. (I have to say that whatever your Marmite views are of Jeremy Clarkson and despite being a cricketing fan of Freddie Flintoff, the programme has never been the same since Clarkson, May and Hammond left). As a result, the three of us had an enjoyable trip in 2012 to *Top Gear Live* at Birmingham NEC.

Perhaps Leah gets her petrol head from me. I have always loved driving, having passed my driving test four months after turning seventeen, and have always been interested in cars. For a while, in the early Nineties, I had a TVR D30 – fun but totally impracticable for someone having no understanding of mechanics. But it was a great car to drive and the engine had a wonderful throaty roar. Once, when pulling away from traffic lights in Aldershot, the roar of the engine made a beat bobby spin round, clearly relishing booking a speeding driver in the middle of the town centre. Instead, he had to give me a disappointing smile as I pootled down the street.

I have been very fortunate in that it soon became evident that Leah shared another of my loves – rock music, and had an inherent aversion to the likes of Justin Bieber or girl groups like Sugarbabes and Girls Aloud, all big in the Noughties. It meant that when she was at an age when she still needed accompanying to concerts, I was not having to sit through interminable bilge!

Vinny did not always attend, but we did go as a family to The O$_2$ for Leah's first concert – the Eagles in 2008. Vinny announced that it was his first concert for thirty-three years. Who had he last seen back in 1975? The Eagles, alongside Elton John and the Beach Boys at Wembley Stadium! He also came with us to see Fleetwood Mac, explaining that the last time he had seen them was at their "farewell" concert at the quaintly named *The Aquae Sulis Incident* at Bath City FC ground in 1970.

Leah quickly progressed to heavy metal and then punk rock (what Vinny termed "shouty shouty f*** f***" music" on the basis that, in his view, all the performers and exponents of this genre ever do is shout and repeat said expletive). I went with Leah to a number of gigs of her choice. One in particular I remember was Black Veil Brides. Whereas I got involved to what, I hope, was a respectable degree with appropriate eye and face make-up, I recall seeing one poor teenager standing and cringing while her comfy dressed father engaged in some awful dad dancing.

On another occasion Vinny had to step in for me as "appropriate adult" when I was called out to a Royal Military Police station in Germany at short notice. He and Leah went, with one of her friends, to Wembley Arena for a four-hour assault on his eardrums, which, as ever, he endured with remarkable good humour and stoicism. He did, however, kick himself afterwards for not doing his homework. It was only on leaving the arena that he discovered Saracens had been playing Harlequins next door at Wembley Stadium and that, with a little bit of smart organisation, he could have accompanied the girls to the concert, slipped out to watch the match, and then returned to collect just before the gig ended. This he always regards as a rare missed opportunity!

Leah has obviously attended many, many gigs now with friends but I am delighted that she still likes to go with me as well. We have seen Bruce Springsteen, the Eagles, Fleetwood Mac and Bryan Adams a number of times, as well as other bands including My Chemical Romance, Mötley Crüe, Whitesnake, Alice Cooper, Guns N' Roses and so on. Vinny remains very selective, joining us for the Eagles, Bruce Springsteen (both occasionally), the Rolling Stones, Madness and Deep Purple.

I am not sure when we will next be able to go to a concert, given both personal and wider societal circumstances. However, given the demographic of the fan base for some of my favourite groups and artists, one of the innovations I am hoping to see before I next attend is the introduction of a mosh pit dedicated to those wearing neck braces!

Another pastime that has tended to be a family affair is visiting the theatre, especially since Leah reached her early teens. But the starting point was not particularly auspicious. When aged about three, Leah went on a nursery trip to the pantomime at the Princes Theatre in Aldershot. As soon as the witches started cackling at the beginning of Act One, Leah began to scream and I had to escort her from the auditorium. As I had volunteered to be one of the drivers ferrying children to and from the theatre, we could not just leave the scene and go home. Instead, we sat out the whole performance in the foyer with a colouring book.

The next visit was a lot more successful in that we went to see the Moscow State Circus perform on stage in Manchester while staying with my sister Kate, who then lived in Lymm, Cheshire. It was a stunning spectacle and Leah was enthralled this time, thus beginning her own love affair with live performance.

When she was a little older, I took her to a matinee performance of *The Lion King* at the Lyceum. Vinny was working and unable to join us, but we did meet for lunch beforehand and watched the street performers in Covent Garden. I shall never forget Leah being transfixed by their antics and the joyous mesmerised look on her face at the Lyceum as the "animals" came down the aisle. I have lost count of how many times she has seen the show since.

Another animal production, *Warhorse*, nearly had us in tears.

Also, at a relatively young age, Leah accompanied us to see *Spamalot* at the Cambridge Theatre. I was in stitches before it even started and can still hear the audience reciting large chunks of Monty Python script in step with the actors. I am glad to say that Leah remains a huge Python fan and has been with us to see *Spamalot* on two further occasions.

Over the years we have seen an eclectic range of momentous performances, including *Twelfth Night* in Stratford-upon-Avon, *Chicago* on Broadway, Omid Djalili as a masterful Fagin in *Oliver Twist*, *Carmen* at the Royal Albert Hall, *Avenue Q*, *Sweeney Todd*, *Les Misérables*, *Miss Saigon* and so on. We enjoyed seeing Peter O'Toole in *Jeffrey Bernard is Unwell* at the Old Vic, where the set was a mock-up of a pub, The Coach and Horses, which was next to Vinny's office when he worked for several years as a VAT inspector in Soho. The proprietor, Norman Balon, advertised himself as the rudest landlord in London (on good evidence) and the *Private Eye* team met weekly in an upstairs room. But I digress!

When Leah became more involved in the selection process, the shows took on a not unsurprising musical flavour. Suddenly we found ourselves going to the likes of *We Will Rock You*, *Rock of Ages*, *The War of the Worlds*, Tina Turner and so on.

Provincial theatres have also featured strongly with visits to Bath, Guildford, Farnham and further afield. We have particularly enjoyed our trips to Richmond Theatre in recent years, with friends Anne and Gary, where we have seen a varied range of shows, always preceded by an excellent meal at the *Pizzeria Rustica*.

It would be wrong of me to omit the odd disappointment, such as the time we went to see *A Tale of Two Cities* on a set consisting of giant sea containers at Regent's Park Open Air Theatre. To say that we found the interpretation of this familiar story hard to follow would be an understatement, and we were just so relieved that rain stopped play before our brains became too scrambled.

On the other hand, in another visit to the Open Air Theatre, we enjoyed a stirring production of *Jesus Christ Superstar*. Declan Bennett's performance as Jesus was outstanding.

Dining out has also featured strongly in our family. A present given to me the first time I had cancer was tea for two at the

Ritz. When we came to book, the only time slot available was 12.30 p.m. so it became lunch for three accompanied by a jazz pianist. Leah, then aged seven, spent much of the time with a look of disdain on her face because of the Chelsea ladies that lunch on the table next to us. They had with them their daughters of similar age to Leah who were overdressed, precocious and badly behaved.

A particularly entertaining dining experience for the three of us was a pre-theatre meal in *Pizza Express* in Covent Garden. Given that it was early evening, there were only a few tables occupied. We selected a booth that contained a small round table for three and a square table for two. As the tables were touching it could also be used as a table for five. To our astonishment two women came in and opted to park themselves on the square table next to us in true 4x4 car-park style. We were momentarily stunned into silence, then discussed among ourselves the psychology that drives some people to herd in open spaces.

They surprisingly complained to us that we were being rude. Leah acerbically pointed out to them that it had been their choice to sit at the table when the restaurant was virtually empty and it had been their choice to then tune in on our conversation. We could not be held responsible if they misinterpreted or did not enjoy what they heard. They promptly moved!

The manager had observed all of this and was so embarrassed that he offered us free desserts.

Many years ago, we went with friends for a meal at *River Cottage* in Fulham. We had specifically booked a table on the outdoor terrace and it was a lovely evening. After we were seated, we were disappointingly moved to an inside table. Once inside, it was explained to us, amid profuse apologies, that our table was a favourite with Woody Allen, who had arrived unannounced, expecting his usual place. Halfway through the evening the heavens opened, by which time all the inside tables were occupied. Poetic justice!

In the early Noughties, we enjoyed doing the rounds of various untried restaurants and gastropubs in and around Hampshire with friends with whom we shared childcare arrangements. The visits were based on personal or media recommendations and resulted in an eclectic range of interesting dining experiences. The nadir was a booking at *The Crown* at Axford, a rural retreat with a strong reputation for fine food and wines. Our visit unfortunately coincided with a perfect storm of proprietors taking a weekend break, an inexperienced relief manager, staff absences, hot weather and an unusually high number of punters arriving on spec, none of whom were turned away. We were seated in the garden due to the weather but, in terms of service, would have fared no worse had we been sitting on picnic chairs in an open field several miles away. Very little on the menu was actually available, food arrived late, cold and incomplete after much chasing, cold drinks were served warm and vice versa and the whole operation had a touch of the *Fawlty Towers* about it. In the end we decided to treat the event as if it were an open-air theatre rather than a restaurant.

But the *pièce de résistance* has to be a trip to Ilfracombe in the mid-Noughties, which was just like stepping back into a Seventies time warp. We lost count of the number of oldies bombing around on their mobility scooters.

Our first attempted lunch stop was a pub. We ordered a round of drinks, then discovered that the only food available was pickled eggs and onions in jars on the bar. As Visa was not acceptable for payment for the drinks, we had to avail ourselves of the cash machine conveniently located in the corner of the bar.

The only restaurant we could find was reminiscent of a post-war sitting room complete with faux multicoloured brick-wall chimney. The menu contained such delights as prawn cocktail, melon balls, pâté and toast or breaded garlic mushrooms for starters; chilli con carne or chicken Kiev for mains; and Black Forest gateau, lemon meringue pie, Arctic Roll or profiteroles for dessert.

Our eventual choices were wheeled out by Mrs Overall's grandmother on a rickety two-tiered tea trolley, crying out for WD40 and identical to the one my mother had in my childhood. The elderly waitress was dressed in a rather faded and badly stained Nippy outfit, presumably bequeathed to her on the closure of the Lyons' Corner Houses. I have to admit by this stage the tears were rolling. Once again cash only – no cheques or cards and we are talking no more than fifteen years ago, at the time of writing!

We have had some wonderful meals in the near vicinity, such as at the *Hotels du Vin* in Winchester and Henley-on-Thames, *L'Ortolan* at Shinfield and Heston Blumenthal's *The Fat Duck* at Bray.

At the latter we opted for the full tasting menu, which included compatible wines for each course. It was a seven-course lunch, with various sub-courses, lasting four hours. One of the courses, flowing with dry ice, was accompanied by sherry, one of my least favourite tipples. I took a sip and turned my nose up. Following a few mouthfuls of the exquisite plate of food in front of me, I automatically took another sip from my glass. What a transformation – delicious. Blumenthal is a true food chemist when it comes to combining flavours.

The range of courses took us through the whole gamut of the day from morning till night, including delicacies such as snail porridge and a liquorice roll accompanied by vodka. We concluded with egg and bacon ice cream – an amazing innovation.

Fine dining experiences do not have to be restricted to top class restaurants. For my mother's eightieth birthday I offered to cook a five-course lunch for eight people. She invited friends from her village, all within walking distance, which was just as well given the state they were in on departure.

I decided to don my chef's jacket (modelled by Vinny the Pinny when he first started cooking after I came out of hospital in March 2020). For the purpose of the occasion, I was accompanied by Vinny the *Sommelier* and Leah the *Maître d'*. Vinny prevailed on me not to sample the wine until preparation of the final course had been completed. This was just as well as I discovered halfway through the meal that one of the guests used to be a professional chef. But my efforts were lauded in a speech at the end by her drunken husband, which was also testament to the sterling work Vinny and Leah had done. I soon caught up for lost time!

In many ways nothing can beat the unexpected, in terms of fine dining, such as breakfast with navvies in *Mother Hubbard's Café* in Kinsale, having just come off the overnight ferry from Swansea, breakfast *bunns* at the famous *Sally Lunn's* in Bath or fish and chips at the *Magpie* in Whitby, sadly burned down the last time we visited.

Returning home to South Warnborough, Hampshire, I can say that because of living in a village with no public transport to speak of, we naturally became taxi drivers for Leah until she passed her test and could drive herself. The journeys we made were many and various, including covering virtually every swimming pool in the south-east of England while she was still into competitive swimming.

There were also some curiosities, including the time Vinny set up "office" in the café at Marwell Zoo while Leah and her friend Rosie, both then aged fifteen, did their own thing. Because both were under sixteen, they had to be accompanied by an adult even though they were mature and responsible. Meanwhile, Vinny had to endure the unruliness and misbehaviour of youngsters in the café allegedly under the control of their parents and guardians. But he got his work done and the girls enjoyed their requested visit so a good result all round.

A taxi memory that we all enjoyed involved a sleepover that Leah spent with a friend in Lychpit, near Basingstoke. Neither Vinny nor I knew the parents beforehand nor where they lived precisely.

Given respective commitments we decided that I would drop off on the Friday afternoon and Vinny would collect on the Saturday. Come the Saturday morning, and using a combination of my directions and satnav, Vinny arrived at the correct spot. As he opened the car door and started peering at numbers on the closely grouped houses, a middle-aged couple literally leapt on him. The conversation went thus.

Mr Gush: "How good to meet you. We were expecting you, of course. Do come in. Do come in."

Vinny: (after being led almost forcibly by the arm into Mr Gush's house and offered a cup of coffee) "No, thank you. I am in a bit of a hurry . . ."

Mr Gush: "In that case we won't detain you . . ." (then proceeding to give a fairly detailed account of how he intends to knock through a wall in the kitchen and move the stairs).

Vinny: (diplomatically) "This is all fascinating and I wish you luck in your endeavours, but as I said I am in a bit of a hurry. If you could therefore slip my daughter from her lair?"

Mr Gush: "Your daughter? But aren't you the interior designer from Homebase?"

Vinny had to explain that he was not and then beat a hasty retreat as Mr Gush tripped over himself, physically and verbally, in a state of acute embarrassment.

At last released from Mr Gush's clutches, Vinny made his way next door to be reunited with Leah and enjoy a good laugh and cup of tea with her friend's parents.

I suppose the moral of this story is not to assume anything, least of all that the man getting out of a BMW near your house is a Homebase interior designer!

At the age of sixteen, Leah embarked on her Duke of Edinburgh (D of E) path. It reminded me of my own experience. I recall that at school we were all issued with booklets enabling us to record our progress through the Bronze Award process.

Unfortunately, that was it. There was no guidance or co-ordinator to assist and we were just expected to get on with it. Consequently, my total contribution to the process was to receive the booklet, open it, look at the blank pages, close it and put it in a drawer. Such strenuous and considered activity!

I am proud to say that Leah achieved markedly more than this. Around the age of fifteen she became an army cadet with a Royal Electrical and Mechanical Engineers unit in Alton. She learned many skills including orienteering which she was able to call upon during her D of E. She could have undertaken the latter with the cadets but opted to do so through her school, Farnborough Hill. She was, nevertheless, able to call on her cadet-acquired skills. One of those skills involved packing a Bergen, which also proved useful later when attending such events as Reading Festival.

Leah was still just sixteen when she achieved her Bronze Duke of Edinburgh Award. There is no requirement to complete Silver before Gold so she opted to move straight to Gold.

This involved a number of elements. First, her four-day orienteering trip took place in the Trossachs near Loch Lomond in Scotland. Rather her than me in the foul weather that settled on the group.

Second, she had to undertake a community project for twelve months. This took the form of spending one afternoon a week in our village with the ailing parents of our friend Jo, thereby enabling Jo to have some respite. Sadly, Jo's parents are no longer with us but I know that Leah has very fond memories of those afternoons.

The third element focused on learning or developing a skill. For this Leah studied for, and passed, grade six on the electric guitar. Bring back 'Smoke on the Water'!

Carrying out a new activity for six months to fulfil the fourth element saw Leah and I attending yoga classes. I have to admit that neither of us lasted a day longer than the required period.

Finally, she had to organise a residential week in a situation completely outside her known comfort zone. To her credit she conducted a considerable amount of research, which resulted in her becoming a student keeper at Blackpool Zoo. Obviously, we had to ferry her there, so rather than make two return trips, we took a cottage for the week in the Forest of Boland. A great time for all of us, although I have to say that I will not be hurrying back to Blackpool itself any day soon.

Consequently, at the age of eighteen she achieved her Gold Award and I went with her (only one guest allowed) to St James's Palace for the presentation by the Duke of Edinburgh himself. A special and proud day out.

In 2016, the sixtieth anniversary of the awards, there was a one-off opportunity to obtain a Diamond Pin by participating in a challenge to raise money for the D of E charity. Leah opted to do a tandem skydive from 15000 feet. Not one for the basophobes!

From Farnborough Hill, Leah went on to the University of Reading for four years before graduating with a degree in Psychology. While there she also managed to fit in some volunteering in Fiji, having also volunteered in Malawi when at school. In Fiji she was involved in redecorating a school to encourage the children to attend and enjoy their education. She also found time to help create pools for baby turtles born on the beach so they could grow in a stable environment and have a better chance of survival. In Malawi the volunteering was focused on the construction of a new school.

Leah was always resourceful in finding paid employment during full-time education, starting with qualification and part-time duties as a lifeguard. Having gone straight from school to university, however, she had always intended to have a gap year on graduating. Sadly, coronavirus put paid to that.

She spent many months volunteering in a food bank in Alton during the early stages of the pandemic and then, despite furlough and restrictions, managed, to her credit, to obtain full-time employment in the hospitality industry (still giving one of her days off to the food bank). Then, at the end of the second lockdown, Leah secured her ideal job in the social housing sector putting to good use some of the skills she learned during her work placement year at University.

We are immensely proud of all that she has achieved. She has also been a great friend and companion. I just hope that as the coronavirus restrictions ease, the full range of opportunities will return, allowing Leah and her generation to continue to exchange enthusiastic endeavour for rich satisfaction and reward.

Returning to Vinny, it was obviously a huge disappointment that a combination of coronavirus and cancer (but mainly the former) prevented him from taking Leah and me to celebrate my sixtieth birthday in August 2020 at the Tom Kerridge pub, *The Hand and Flowers*, in Marlow, Buckinghamshire, as originally planned and booked.

Ever since we have been together, he has gone to great lengths to ensure that my significant birthdays are celebrated in memorable style. When I turned forty, on 16 August 2000, Vinny took me to the OXO Tower in London, a wonderful experience enhanced by the view over the Thames through the full glass wall. We had opted for an early evening booking. Unexpected entertainment was provided during our starters by a table of drunken city slickers finishing off their lunch that had clearly been largely liquid-based.

A month later I experienced the rest of my wonderful birthday present that Vinny had created by drawing together all my interests – art, travel, sport, gardening, history, reading and, of course, alcohol! We travelled by car to Giverny, France, for the weekend, taking with us a new book that Vinny had bought me, entitled *A Social History of English Cricket*, and a forty-year-old bottle of port, having been told at Berry Bros. & Rudd that 1960 was a crap year for wine!

Monet's Garden did not disappoint and, amazingly, we had the place to ourselves. But the garden itself only brought together art, travel and gardening. We still had to weave in the other interests. This we did by decanting the port into a vessel suitable for smuggling before heading off for the famous bridge spanning the water lilies. Once there I was able to take a few surreptitious sips while learning more about the social history of cricket and taking in the splendid sights before me. Never before – or since – have I been able to combine my principal leisure interests in a single moment! An extraordinary birthday celebration indeed!

It seems strange, looking back, that cancer had the audacity to visit me between my fortieth and fiftieth birthdays and, not being satisfied, decided to return to leave its indelible mark between the ages of fifty and sixty. But it takes more than an intervention by the Big C to spoil my fun or dampen my spirits!

10

Rugby Geek

Vinny has always enjoyed explaining to friends and colleagues that his wife loves sport and hates shopping. And it is true. As I mentioned earlier, I have never particularly excelled at physical participation. But that has never stopped me trying, nor being an avid spectator.

My strong preference is for rugby in the winter and cricket in the summer, and to attend to support my favourite teams rather than slump in front of the television. However, the gradual erosion of the traditional breaks between winter and summer sports, the changes to start times and dates demanded by TV scheduling, and the plethora of international matches played globally all year round, have combined to present quite a significant logistical challenge to ardent spectators in the modern age. Consequently, a subscription to satellite sports channels has become as much of a necessity for us diehards as an annual season ticket. The former certainly proved their worth as major sports were reduced to being played behind closed doors during the Covid-19 restrictions.

My love for both rugby and cricket undoubtedly came from my father, although my mother has always enjoyed cricket and tennis – in reverse order! I first started watching rugby with my father as a child. The focus was the Five Nations on BBC Television (before it became the Six Nations with the admission of Italy in 2000), and I soon gained an understanding of the laws (not rules!) of the game sitting alongside him.

One of those Five Nations games really sticks in my mind. It was a particularly violent encounter at Twickenham between England and Wales, which ended in a narrow England victory by nine points to eight. The Welsh flanker Paul Ringer was red-carded during the game. The match was only about ten minutes old when the referee had to warn both captains that if they could not control their players, somebody would be leaving the field. A couple of minutes later Ringer was guilty of a late tackle, followed by injudicious use of the elbow . . . and off he trotted. To again quote an overused modern cliché, lessons should have been learned. Clearly, they had not been.

One of the joys of attending a live rugby match is that there is rarely any animosity between opposing fans. As a result, there is no segregation in the grounds, nor in the pubs and surrounding areas before and after the games. This means that fans, including family groups, are able to travel to away fixtures, donning club shirts and scarves, safe in the knowledge that they will not encounter any unpleasantness. On the contrary, it is probable that they will meet supporters from the opposing side and be able to engage in good-humoured conversation about the game we all love.

Travelling to away grounds for European club fixtures is particularly special as it provides the opportunity to combine two pleasure-pursuits in the form of live sport and sightseeing. Although I have to admit that at times it can be extremely frustrating being a travelling supporter. Vinny and I are Bath Rugby season-ticket holders and in the 2019/20 season, before it was interrupted by Covid-19, we lost all six of our European group-stage games, both home and away. Taking in the sights on a city break can usually be extremely enjoyable, but slightly less so in deepest December or January when your team has been on the end of yet another drubbing!

But the prospect of an embarrassing defeat has never been sufficient to deter us from planning an away trip to support the Blue, Black and Whites, and explore the main tourist attractions, wherever the luck of the European draw might take us.

Focussing on more recent seasons, in April 2017 we spent a weekend in Paris to see Bath play away to *Stade Français* in a European Challenge Cup semi-final. Having been to Paris many times, we tried to visit attractions that we had not seen before, such as the *Panthéon* and *Sainte-Chapelle*. But we could not resist old favourites such as the *Musée d'Orsay* and the *Louvre* for a special Vermeer exhibition.

On the morning of the match, we walked several miles from our hotel close to the *Stade Jean-Bouin* along the banks of the Seine to the centre of Paris. It was a bright, crisp morning and we rounded off the invigorating walk with a splendid light lunch. We then came back down to earth by watching Bath snatch defeat from the jaws of victory, to deny themselves a place in the final in Edinburgh – for which we had tickets. Oh well!

In December 2017 we travelled to Nice for an away fixture in the European Champions Cup at Toulon, a two-hour train ride away. The benefit of travelling at this time of year is the dearth of tourists, combined with the ability to book city centre hotels at reasonable cost. Similar to Clermont a year later, there was an excellent Christmas market a mere stone's throw from the hotel, from where we could also look out over the Mediterranean.

As we were due to leave Nice, Storm Clara swept in, forcing

the airport to close, resulting in us enjoying two extra nights courtesy of British Airways. Looking back, I would like to think that the unexpected free extension compensated for the frustrating Bath defeat by Toulon. But the sad fact is that it did not!

On a happier note, from both a travel and rugby result perspective, we spent a memorable weekend in Venice in January 2018, from where we took a train ride to Treviso for the away fixture with Benetton. On arrival in Venice city centre, by water taxi from the airport, we were most grateful to have Google Maps on our phones in order to successfully wend our merry way through the myriad of tiny lanes to our hotel. That turned out to be an absolute delight, with our room having a rooftop terrace overlooking the Grand Canal.

As with the trip to Nice in the previous month, the beauty of travelling to Venice in the depths of winter was that all the attractions were open but visitor numbers were at a seasonal low. We travelled by boat to all of the islands, managed to visit numerous historic buildings and museums and feasted on the delights of Italian cuisine. Venice is a beautiful city and it is such a shame to think of it sinking. Who in their right minds can continue to deny climate change and its devastating impact!

To add gloss to a memorable weekend, Bath Rugby did us proud by defeating Benetton in Treviso and narrowly missing out on a quarter final place in the European Champions Cup.

On another rugby-themed weekend, we flew to Dublin in December 2018 to see Bath play away to Leinster at the Aviva Stadium. As with the two previous trips, and those mentioned later, the competition was once again the European Champions Cup. Apart from watching the rugby and doing some sightseeing, we thought it might provide us with a welcome break from the constant talk of Brexit in the home news. Sadly, there was no escape because the taxi drivers insisted on talking about nothing else and interrogating us about the rationale behind the decision to leave the EU. I am afraid that we were searching for the same answers ourselves so could not help them on that one!

In between the Brexit discussions we managed to fit in visits to Kilmainham Gaol with its fascinating information about political prisoners; the National Gallery of Ireland; Dublin Castle; and Christ Church Cathedral, where we experienced a joyous Christmas concert. We still, of course, left ourselves time to partake of some libations in Temple Bar.

Oh, I almost forgot. Bath Rugby suffered a heavy defeat at the hands of Leinster!

January 2019 found us in Toulouse. This provided a good example of being led to a city you might not otherwise visit in isolation by following the fortunes of your favourite sports team.

We entered the impressive *Basilique Saint-Sernin, Couvent des Jacobins* and the fine arts museum, the *Musée des Augustins*, all well worth their place on any sightseeing trail. We stayed in a central hotel on the *Place du Capitole.*

Unfortunately, while we were there, the *Gilet Jaune* protests were in full swing. It was later reported on the news stream, *Somerset Live*, that Bath supporters had been caught up in the riots. We managed to skirt round them and only had to suffer the smell of tear gas in our nostrils. Needless to say, Bath Rugby lost the ensuing game to Toulouse!

Eleven months later saw us heading off to Clermont-Ferrand for the fourth group stage game against Clermont

Auvergne on 15 December 2019. This time we were fortunate enough to be able to bag seats on the team's charter flight from Bristol. As we were approaching our destination the captain announced, "I should warn you that the descent into Clermont is likely to be extremely bumpy. This is because our normal weight distribution has been compromised by the entire Bath Rugby team sitting up front!"

Being December the Christmas market was in full swing and the atmosphere in the town was electrifying. The Clermont fans were most welcoming, including a group enjoying a street party who insisted that we join in and partake of their wine.

Oh yes, there was another game of rugby; this time we lost 52-26 to go with the 17-34 defeat at home against the same team the previous week. But Clermont's stadium was magnificently atmospheric, and it was a fascinating experience to be able to travel with the team and enjoy drinks with the CEO, Tarquin McDonald, and Director of Rugby, Stuart Hooper and the rest of the coaching staff in the hotel reception the evening before the game.

Our final trip before the Covid pandemic and cancer rudely interrupted involved a delightful visit to Belfast in January 2020. Having lost at home to Ulster by a narrow margin in the opening 2019/20 group fixture, the return at Ulster's Kingspan Stadium for the last of the six group games was always going to be a tricky affair.

Flying into Belfast International can be hairy to say the least, even for a lover of air travel like me, because of the crosswinds. But on this occasion we landed without incident and within an hour we were exploring the fascinating *Titanic Experience*, which opened in 2012 in the spectacularly rejuvenated Titanic Quarter.

Over the weekend we also managed to fit in a black cab political tour of the Falls and Shanklin Road areas, taking in Crumlin Gaol and the Peace Wall, plus a trip around the Antrim coast that included a walk on the Giant's Causeway, followed by some delightful light refreshment at the Old Bushmills Distillery. Oh yes, there was also a game of rugby that Bath lost, but in a game that the 22–15 scoreline indicates was more even than we anticipated.

Apart from the result it was a thoroughly enjoyable weekend, even allowing for the fact that, for the ninth month in a row, I was travelling around unaware that I was riddled with cancer and with a disconnect between my neck and the rest of my spine!

My stories of Bath Rugby consistently losing European away games we have attended in recent seasons are not told in a critical fashion. We have almost become immune to being on the wrong end of a poor outcome. As the rugby correspondent and former Bath player, David Flatman, once commented it is a club that has under-delivery built into its DNA! The important thing is that our weekends have not been spoiled by the results, nor have our spirits been dampened. On the domestic front we have also travelled the length and breadth of England, visiting all the current Premiership grounds, together with some that are now home to Championship sides. In the course of such travels, we have enjoyed seeing many a Bath win on the road. We will continue to follow Bath with a passion and, my physical challenges allowing, fit in as many European away fixtures as we possibly can.

As already indicated, the 2019/20 season was disappointingly, but understandably, disrupted in March 2020 by Covid-19. This occurred at around the same time that I received my cancer diagnosis, along with news about the related damage to my neck and other bones. Indeed, I watched the last pre-lockdown home match against Bristol on 1 March 2020 in some considerable pain, I must admit, before visiting the Royal National Orthopaedic Hospital in Stanmore on 6 March 2020 for a private consultation to seek the second opinion. It was during the penultimate round of pre-lockdown televised matches, between Bristol and Harlequins on 8 March 2020, that my consultant telephoned to hint at bad news and the need for urgent tests. Then, of course, I received the unwelcome diagnosis back at Stanmore on 11 March 2020.

The absence of live rugby, both at the Recreation Ground and on television, left a big, strange hole in our lives during the early months of the first Covid-19 lockdown. It was therefore with great relief and jubilation that the green light was given for the season to recommence in August 2020 under new, Covid-19-influenced conditions, including the absence of spectators.

The performance of Bath Rugby on their return to competitive rugby was well worth the wait, with seven wins, one draw and one narrow loss in the nine Gallagher Premiership games that were left in the season, finishing in fourth place and earning a semi-final play-off place in the process. Sadly, their route to the final was blocked by a strong Exeter Chiefs side who triumphed 35-6 on their home turf.

The disappointment felt at being unable to attend the Rec due to the Covid-19 pandemic was exacerbated on one particular occasion when we were lucky enough to be drawn in a ballot of season-ticket holders to attend the home game against Gloucester in the early evening of Tuesday 22 September 2020. The club had gone to considerable lengths to ensure a safe environment for the 1,000 supporters permitted to attend on a pilot basis.

On a personal level I was between the first and second phases of my treatment plan, feeling in good shape and satisfied that attending the Rec presented no threats or dangers. Then within a matter of hours before kick-off, the Government inexplicably pulled the plug as it prepared for a potential second spike that was emerging in the north of the country. In keeping with the Government's often illogical and inconsistent handling of the Covid-19 pandemic, the last-minute decision to ban spectators from attending meant that it would not be possible to watch the game in a strictly controlled open space, prepared with meticulous precision, but possible to decamp to less secure confined spaces in local city centre pubs to watch the game on television.

We were left exasperated by the sudden and incomprehensible *volte-face*, but at least we had not yet set off on our ninety-mile journey to the ground, suitably equipped to remain self-sufficient in our specially constructed social bubble for at least eight hours!

Sadly, due to the Covid-19 restrictions, virtually the whole of the 2020/21 season was played behind closed doors. Fortunately, we were among the 3,000 loyal season-ticket holders allowed into the ground to watch the final game on 12 June 2021.

After driving Miss Issy to our allocated disabled spot in the ground, Vinny escorted me to a seat outside a city centre pub where we soaked up the atmosphere surrounded by fellow fans, just so happy to be back. It was amazing how different the city looked in the glorious sunshine when we were so used to being there in the freezing cold and/or torrential rain.

Once in the ground we had our customary pasty before the match started. Oh, I have never enjoyed a pasty so much! We went on to win an enjoyable but nerve-racking game with the highlight being a sixty-five-yard unchallenged run down the pitch by Josh Bayliss, roared on by the crowd, to score a try with the clock in the red. The win ensured European Champions Cup Rugby for the 2021/22 season.

The afternoon ended with the squad doing a lap of honour round the pitch. Some were accompanied by their young children. I will not deny becoming emotional. By rights I should not have been at the match given my initial prognosis. But I will not be beaten. And in September 2021 I was back at the Rec for the new season in our upgraded seats, specifically chosen to enable me to watch the flow of the game without having to constantly move my head (one of the consequences of wearing a neck brace is that I can no longer move my head without moving the rest of my upper body. Sadly activities, such as rubbernecking, are now just a distant memory!)

It was in the early stages of my illness that I began to realise that the special relationship that flows from being a member of the Bath Rugby family extends far beyond the focal point of what happens on the pitch at the heart of a UNESCO World Heritage site. The club has been incredibly supportive of my situation since first hearing in May 2020 about my diagnosis.

Much to my surprise and delight, I received a personal and fairly lengthy video message from the Bath Rugby CEO,

Tarquin McDonald, whom Vinny and I have had the pleasure to meet over drinks in both Toulouse and Clermont-Ferrand.

Tarquin said that he had heard that I had been doing "crazy things" like travelling to rugby matches with a broken neck and, in wishing me well, said that he admired my typically female resilience – in a very self-deprecating way.

This was followed by a second video message, this time from the Bath Director of Rugby, Stuart Hooper. In addition to expressing his concern and best wishes in very warm and sincere terms, Stuart invited Vinny and I down to their magnificent training facilities at Farleigh House to have lunch with him and some of the players when Covid-19 restrictions allow.

Both wonderful gestures that brought a smile to my face and a small tear to my eye. I obviously sent suitable responses, including an acceptance of the invitation.

If that was not enough, a month later I received another wonderful surprise from Bath Rugby in the shape of a personal video message from their captain and England international, Charlie Ewells. It was a message delivered with genuine warmth and empathy, and serves to underline just what a close-knit and caring club Bath Rugby is to support and be a proud member of.

Our rugby-related travels have not been restricted to following Bath. We have also enjoyed European finals weekends, having booked tickets and made the necessary travel arrangements well before it was known who would be competing.

European Premiership Rugby holds its top and second tier cup finals on the same weekend in the same European city, selected annually to ensure that the game gets the widest possible exposure across the continent.

In May 2018 it was the turn of Bilbao. Spain is not a country where you would expect to watch top-flight rugby union, nor is Bilbao a city that you would think of as being on the main tourist trail. But we had a fantastic long weekend, the highlights being a visit to the magnificent Guggenheim Art Museum and a trip out to San Sebastian for a private walking and taxi tour. We learned much about Basque history and cuisine in the process.

Undoubtedly, our most amazing rugby trip was to Japan in September and October 2019 to follow England in the World Cup. Looking back, I do not know how I managed to spend twenty-eight days touring Japan with a broken neck, but I was determined not to allow what I thought was just a little pain to prevent me from making the most of such a once-in-a-lifetime trip.

We started by flying from Heathrow to Sapporo on the northern island of Hokkaido, via Hong Kong, for the opening England group stage game against Tonga.

Apart from visiting the delightful botanical gardens and viewing the TV tower, we wandered through the Autumn Fest and rugby fanzone before calling in at the beer museum. Outside the museum we met some Australian fans who were in the city for their game against Fiji. They wanted to gloat about their win to a Pommy audience, so Vinny's suggestion that Australia had only won because the captain, like his cricketing counterpart, had rubbed the ball with sandpaper, did not go down at all well and they soon disappeared.

Both the Australian and England games were played at the amazing Sapporo Dome stadium with the roof closed. As

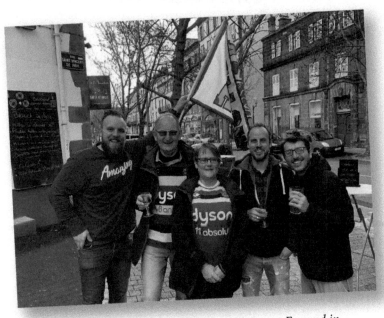

Street party with French fans in Cleremont-Ferrand in December 2019

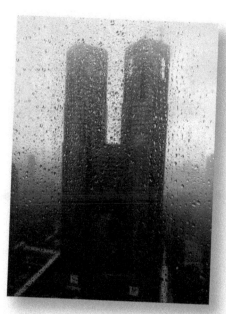

Watching Typhoon Hagibis from the 45th floor of our Tokyo hotel in October 2019

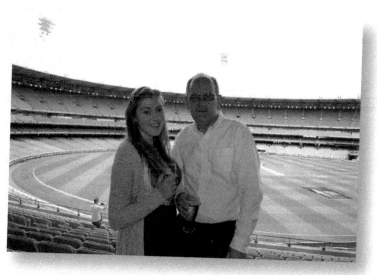

*Vinny and Leah at Melbourne Cricket Ground on
Christmas Day 2013*

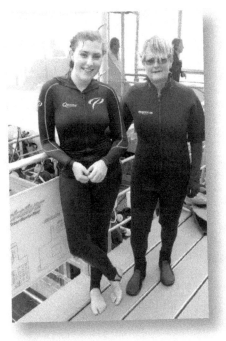

*Preparing to Scuba
Dive on the Great
Barrier Reef, Australia
in January 2014*

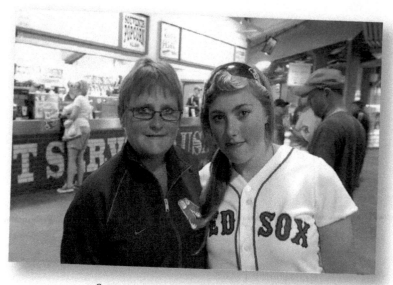

Supporting the Red Sox at Fenway Park,
Boston in July 2012

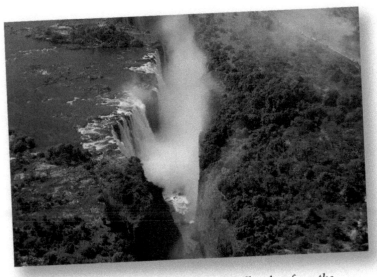

Our helicopter view of the Victoria Falls taken from the
Zambian side in July 2013

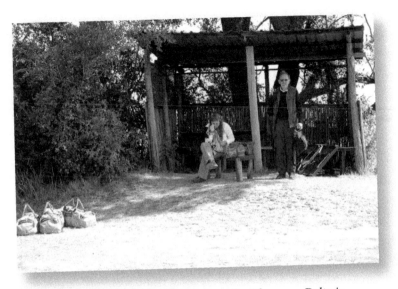

Arrivals and Departure lounge at the Okavango Delta in August 2013

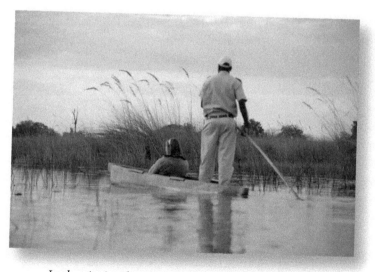

Leah enjoying the rigours of mokoro transportation in the Okavango Delta in August 2013

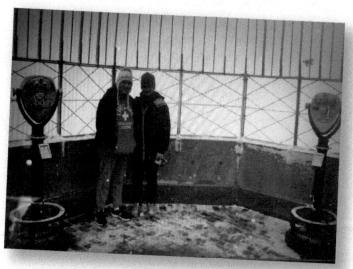

*"Don't you guys know there is zero visibility up
there?" Defying the guides to reach the Empire
State Building viewing platform. February 2007*

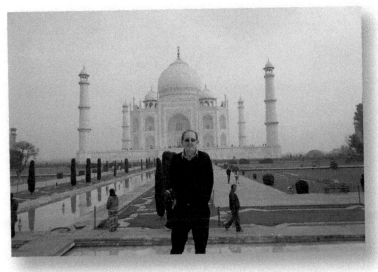

*Vinny's poor attempt to outdo all previous portraits taken
in front of the Taj Mahal, India. February 2012*

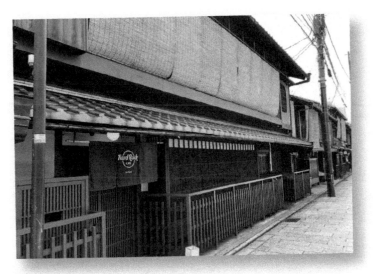

The most untypical Hard Rock Café I have visited.
Kyoto, Japan. October 2019

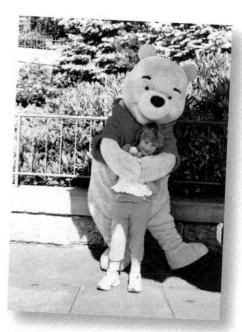

Leah meets Pooh
Bear at Paris
Disney in June
2001

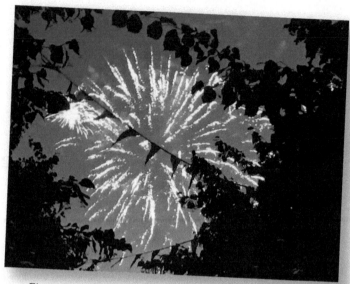

Fireworks at Hampton Court Flower Show to mark the end of RHS members' pre-view day. July 2018

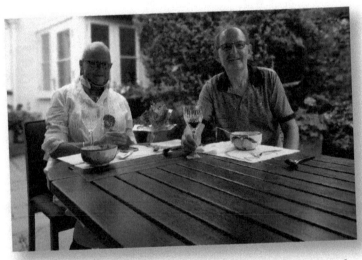

Celebrating my 60th birthday at home in Covid lockdown mode with a post chemo glass of something strong. August 2020

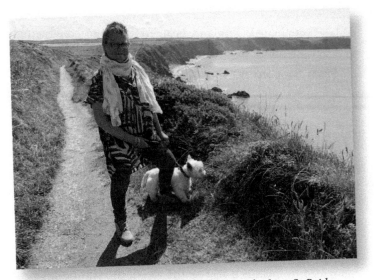

On the Pembrokeshire Coastal Path overlooking St Brides Bay in July 2021

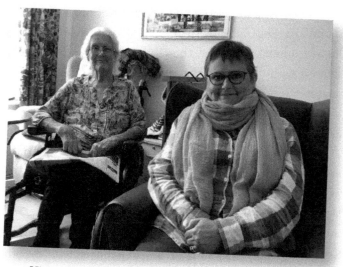

Visiting mother at her residential care home for the first time in sixteen months, following the rude interruptions of Covid and my cancer treatment. June 2021

widely anticipated, England beat Tonga quite convincingly and so were off to the start they needed.

From Sapporo we flew to Osaka on the main island of Honshu. As our plane pushed back from its stand, it was a cultural eye-opener to watch the ground crew standing in a line and bowing simultaneously towards us.

Once in our Osaka hotel we met some more Australians. We relayed Vinny's exchange outside the beer museum in Sapporo and their countrymen's surprisingly negative reaction. Our new Queensland friends helpfully explained "Aww spit, they must have been from Sydney."

We only had one full day of sightseeing in Osaka but managed to include a trip to the top of the stunning Umeda Sky Tower with its views across the city. No *basophobia* problems encountered there.

From Osaka we moved on to Kobe, overlooked by magical mountain ranges, and with amazing harbour views from our high-rise hotel. However, the city was tinged with a certain sadness with its earthquake-memorial shrines relating to the devastation wreaked in 1995 when around 6,000 people were killed, 40,000 injured, 300,000 displaced and $200 billion of damage caused.

While in Kobe we took ourselves off on the local Japanese rail service to Himenji, Japan's first world heritage site. There we saw a fabulous example of a shogun castle and surrounding Japanese garden. More bizarrely, on the morning of moving on from Kobe, we observed out of our hotel window what appeared to be a large open-air market that had not been there on other mornings. On closer inspection we discovered that it was a canine market selling all sorts of items that any respecting owner might wish to purchase for their pooch – delightful clothing outfits, wheelie buggies to carry them around in, and vegan food stalls. The punters were wheeling their charges around in an array of carts; in one we saw six Yorkshire terriers, all with matching hair ribbons. Each to their own.

As to the main reason for being in Kobe, England duly beat the USA without too much difficulty at the imposing Kobe Misaki Stadium. Two games down and two to go – or so we thought.

Our next stop was Kyoto, the former capital of Japan. Here the Imperial Palace and gardens were magical, as was the Nijo castle. With its numerous but contrasting Buddhist temples and Shinto shrines, it is little wonder that the city is one of Japan's foremost tourist attractions.

While in Kyoto we also took the Shinkansen, the bullet train, to Hiroshima. We wandered through the moving Peace Memorial Park from which we could observe the only remaining damaged structure from the 1945 nuclear bombing. Not surprisingly, it is known as the A-Bomb Dome.

We also visited the Peace Memorial Museum for an emotional roller-coaster ride, generated by the juxtaposition of exhibits that spark deep distress with those that instil enormous admiration and optimism.

The day concluded with a bus, then ferry ride to Miyajima Island to visit the stunning Itsukushima Shrine, located in picturesque surroundings just off the shoreline.

Our next stop in following the England rugby team around Japan was Kanazawa, where we were fortunate enough to visit the castle, Samurai house, the Kenroku-en Japanese gardens and geisha district during the course of three days.

On departing from Kanazawa, we took another Shinkansen for our final city-stay in Tokyo. The efficiency of the Shinkansen trains is mightily impressive. Only thirty seconds are allowed at each station for passengers to embark and disembark. When initially informed of this the natural reaction is to panic, particularly if, like me, one has had a lifetime's experience of travelling with SWR or GWR in the south of England. But the process is so fine-tuned and clear. Each ticket tells you exactly where to stand on the platform. The train arrives. Doors open. Passengers get off and on without issue and everything runs like clockwork. If only I could have brought back to the UK this example of Japanese superiority with me!

Tokyo was a whole new ball game (excuse the pun)! Due to the size of the city and the traffic congestion, we stayed at three different hotels. Our first hotel was in the Shinagawa district with its charming waterfront location. From there we attended the Ajinomoto Stadium, also known as the Tokyo Stadium, where we saw a tense game against Argentina. The atmosphere was electric and England won again, helped to a small degree by the indiscipline of their opponents, who had a player sent off for a reckless challenge.

Thereafter we enjoyed a further eight days of sightseeing across the sprawling city before the final scheduled group game against France. That proved an extremely busy time.

We took a trip out of the city to see Mount Fuji. Unfortunately, she did not want to see us. We discovered that there are relatively few days in a year when you can get a clear view because of the predominantly low cloud. Instead, we found ourselves sailing across Lake Ashi in the shadow of the shrouded Mount Fuji on a Hakone pirate ship!

Another fascinating day was spent strolling through the off-the-beaten tourist track through the older Yanessen district to Ueno Park. We passed through the huge Yanaka Cemetery, enjoyed light refreshment in Kabaya Coffee, a café in a 100-year-old traditional Japanese house, before arriving in the park, which contains, among others, the Tokyo National Museum, the National Museum for Western Art and the Metropolitan Art Museum.

Our second hotel was on the Daiba man-made island with its wonderful views over Tokyo Bay and the Rainbow Bridge. The island is 3.2 metres above sea level, which Vinny described as "Canary Wharf on steroids". From our hotel we could walk into the Shiokaze Park where it had been intended to set up a temporary venue for the beach volleyball events for the 2020 Olympics before they too fell victim, temporarily at least, to the Covid-19 pandemic.

As we arrived at our third hotel, in the Shinjuku district, we bumped into the England team, who were leaving for their next location. We all milled around in the foyer wishing them well for the rest of the tournament. You would not be able to do that with the England football team, I suspect.

Also present were a number of Scottish fans, a drunken one of whom decided – unwisely – that it might be a good idea to take Vinny on verbally. During the remonstrations by the fan, who was clearly spoiling for a fight, Vinny sussed him out as being ex-military. Questions about his former unit and advice about my work in courts martial led the fan mistakenly to believe that I was a prosecutor. We will never know what dark secrets he may have been hiding in his past, but he quickly became spooked, abruptly dropped his vain attempts to draw

Vinny into combat, and scarpered without trace.

We spent the next few days trying to live the life of a Tokyoite on a rare home vacation. As we had a total of eight days in Tokyo, and three still remained after our final hotel move, there was certainly no need to rush. We focused the rest of the time on the central areas, with time allocated to strolling through the districts of Shinjuku, including its equivalent of Soho – Roppongi – where we found a safe refuge for my seafood allergy (a Hard Rock Cafe); and Shibuya where the famous square is criss-crossed by numerous zebra crossings. The vehicular traffic from every direction is stopped at the same time, allowing as many as 2,500 pedestrians to cross at the same time.

As the week progressed, concerns grew about Typhoon Hagibis, which was gradually building strength in the Pacific ready for a full-frontal assault on the Japanese mainland. Although the precise timing, course and impact were difficult to predict, they were sufficiently accurate to cause England's final group game against France on 12 October 2019 in Yokohama to be cancelled on safety grounds. From a pure rugby perspective, this brought our tour to a premature, disappointing and rather anticlimactic end. But it proved the right decision, and our disappointment melted into insignificance when compared with the death and destruction that Hagibis caused when it eventually hit landfall.

In a somewhat surreal moment, the group of supporters that had been destined to travel together to Yokohama for England's match against France, headed instead for the forty-fifth floor of our tower block hotel to take part in a pub quiz. It was a quintessentially British scene, with the building gently swaying as it was buffeted by the mighty typhoon in the pitch-black of the afternoon, while contestants inside engaged in heated argument about the nationality of Mata Hara! I cannot recall who won, or what the prizes were.

We had been due to travel back to the UK the following day, but Narita International Airport was closed due to Typhoon Hagibis. We were therefore obliged to stay an extra three nights courtesy of Gullivers Travels and Cathay Pacific. What a shame!

While we were able to relax for a further three days, the tournament officials and administrators were left to determine the fate of outstanding fixtures disrupted by Hagibis, and ensure that the group stages concluded in a fair and equitable fashion.

Luckily, England and France had already qualified for the quarterfinals. While, therefore, we would have dearly loved to see England battle it out against our old adversary for the top-of-group-table bragging rights, at least our progression to the next phase of the tournament was unaffected.

Travelling around Tokyo on public transport had been a relative breeze. I did occasionally struggle with the numerous flights of stairs on the metro because of a marked lack of escalators but, again, that might have had something to do with my unbeknownst broken neck. There were no language problems because all the metro lines and stations were also written using the Roman alphabet, all public announcements were in both Japanese and English, metro and street maps were frequent, and whenever we stopped to scratch our heads, we were pounced on by locals offering to help. Payment was by use of an Oyster card equivalent. There was no need to try and calculate how much we needed to top up the cards because, at the end of our time, we simply handed the cards in and received a cash refund of the unused balance. Another lesson for our own train services in the UK!

To us it seemed that the Rugby World Cup, while a major tournament coup in itself for the Japanese, was in fact a dry run for the 2020 Olympics and Paralympics. An incredible amount of new building and regeneration was taking place. What a shame that Covid-19 intervened in such a cruel way.

The only troublesome matter we encountered in Japan related to food. As previously mentioned, I have an allergy to shellfish and was warned at the outset of the trip that the Japanese do not deal with such issues in the way we do, and there was a strong possibility of cross-contamination.

During the time we were there, we joined a number of organised day trips that usually included lunch in a typically local restaurant. To start with I would just watch the others eat, but soon concluded that lunch consumption made for a pretty boring spectator sport so we skipped them altogether. On one such occasion we found ourselves in a drab business district with little sign of finding food and drink suitable for our needs. We wandered into a small, traditional takeaway and managed to communicate that we would like to purchase two beers. The shop owner produced a little table and two chairs and signalled for us to sit in the tiny serving area of the shop. He disappeared we know not where and returned after a short interval with four cans of beer. He then went into his kitchen and reappeared with a stunning plate of delicacies that, embarrassingly, we could not eat because of my allergy concerns. He could not have done more for us – all for the princely sum of Y300 (about £2). Such hospitality.

Because of my seafood allergy we relied heavily on buying

our food from the ubiquitous 7-Eleven stores (with a heavy focus on egg sandwiches and various salads). We supplemented these main staples with the occasional visit to a Hard Rock Café, Sizzler or an Italian restaurant depending on what we could find. Given the nature of my dietary constraints in a country deeply devoted to all things seafood, the alternative arrangements we made really did work to a tee and I was able to return home unscathed and, to my delight, a half-stone lighter. The only time I have ever lost weight while on holiday!

All of that said, we did take a slight risk by joining our group's final night dinner at a very smart but traditional Japanese restaurant. It had typical floor-level bench seating with leg room created in the sunken cavity under the table. On the basis of my experience over the previous four weeks, I knew I could be selective about the food and survive.

Another notable occurrence came about at the end of the evening. A rather large and drunken British woman got up to leave from a nearby table, stumbled and fell over Vinny's shoulder directly into his lap. Vinny took it in magnanimous style (despite whispering a complaint to the waiter that this was not what he had ordered). She was very embarrassed!

So ended a truly memorable trip of a lifetime to the Rugby World Cup in Japan in the autumn of 2019. It is rather alarming to think that I would not have been able to undertake the tour had I been diagnosed beforehand with the pre-existing cancer and broken neck. Admittedly, I did suffer some pain during those four weeks and relied on a mixture of heat pads and painkillers to keep me going at times. But as Vinny will testify, I found no reason to complain while there nor withdraw from any activities. I embarked on the tour as a fanatical rugby geek and came back with my reputation as such enhanced! If I could change anything, looking back, it would be the result in the final tie between England and South Africa and my absence from that alternative, fantasy game!

II

Cricket Nerd with Extras

Alongside rugby union, cricket has provided me with much enjoyment on the sporting front over many years. I first became interested in the game as a small child. During the Sixties, before the advent of BBC 2, Wimbledon fortnight was televised on the only BBC channel then available. My mother would plant the ironing board in front of the television to watch tennis, tennis and more tennis. It opened up a different world for me to that provided by *Watch with Mother* as children's television was taken off the menu in the Dailley household.

Transmission in the second week was shared with the Lord's Test match and that is how I learned to appreciate the game. My father also umpired frequently for our local team. He loved the game and would have liked to play but was unable to do so because of the polio he contracted during the Second World War.

When I was going out with Julian in the late Seventies, he played for Fyfield Cricket Club, a local team near Windsor. I was expected, along with other wives and girlfriends, to offer my fair share of time in preparing the teas. I was a bit disgruntled about this as I much preferred to watch the cricket. However, I soon discovered that scorers were in very short supply. Much to the delight of the club I offered to learn the cricket scorer's art. A win-win situation. The club had a scorer and I got out of making the teas.

I became a bit of a pedant with my scoring technique, using

different coloured pencils for each bowler, thereby enabling the players, if they were so inclined, to note which batsmen had taken runs off which bowlers. However, I have never taken this obsession to its extreme by turning up at a county or international match with scorebook and pencils tucked under my arm and devoting the entire day to watching and recording every ball!

In my experience, spectators at cricket matches are, generally speaking, far quirkier than those who attend games of rugby. Consequently, *people-watching* offers a rich source of alternative viewing for cricket lovers, and could almost be classed as a secondary attraction that is well worth the entrance fee in its own right.

Participating in this byplay also helps to spot and avoid those individuals who, although extremely well meaning, possess an innate and uncanny ability to spoil one's day at the drop of a hat. In reminiscing with Vinny, during the first Covid-19-induced lockdown in 2020, we soon began to appreciate the lessons we had learned about social distancing through cricket spectatorship – without appreciating just how valuable they would become in the eye of a pandemic.

When heading off to watch a cricket match and landing in unfamiliar terrain, we have tended to forgo Google Maps and other technological aids, in favour of simply tracking the local cricket fanatic to ensure direct passage to the ground. Such fanatics are easily identifiable in their faux Hush Puppies, crumpled chinos flying at half mast through excessive wear and washing, Hawaiian shirts, floppy, grubby sun hats festooned with badges and other cricket memorabilia, Poundland-branded cool boxes, canvas rucksacks still inked with legends of yesteryear, such as Peters and Lee or Mott the

Hoople, autograph books and the cricket equivalent of Michael Portillo's *Bradshaw's Guide – Wisden Cricketer's Almanack* and *Playfair Cricket Annual.*

It is important to keep one's distance from these particular fanatics, not because they are unpleasant or difficult – far from it. The problem is that getting close means the risk of engaging in conversation that, for the sake of comfort and credibility, requires a level of knowledge including topics such as the precise nature of the knee injury that caused Denis Compton to limp but still score centuries, towards the end of 1947. It also encompasses the ability to recite the number of every living Test player aged over 80 in alphabetical order; and to explain the intricacies of DLS to a visiting Martian. (DLS being the Duckworth-Lewis-Stern method, which is a mathematical formulation designed to calculate the target score for the team batting second in a limited-overs match interrupted by weather or other circumstance.) I have yet to meet anyone beyond the fanatical diehards who can explain how it works. Only cricket could require such a complex system.

Once safely escorted to the ground by our willing but unsuspecting Mr Anorak, the fun really begins as we face the challenges presented by the vagaries of organisational competence and customer care for which the cricket authorities are universally renowned. Not to mention those spectators whose primary purpose in attending is to consume vast quantities of alcohol rather than watch the game.

On arrival, we decide to allow Mr Anorak to enter via a different gate to find the same seat he has occupied for the past forty years, partake of the first of his shrimp paste and cucumber sandwiches, pour a cup of Camp coffee from his trusty flask, open a new page in his fading scorebook and sharpen his coloured pencils.

Our next task is to negotiate our way past Mr Stasi the security guard and his unsophisticated but forceful interrogation. I manage to satisfy him that my designer handbag does not contain a false bottom, that I have not decanted a bottle of *Château Mouton Rothschild 1945* into my Robert Dyas Thermos. Obviously, I would never dream of smuggling in alcohol when, inside the ground, I will have *carte blanche* to consume as much alcohol as I wish at four times the fair market price.

Having got past this hurdle it is now time to subject ourselves to the idiosyncrasies of the cricket authorities and their Basil Fawltyesque service standards. Here is a world where it is seen as a privilege to have been allowed to enter their hallowed premises, regardless of cost, and be subjected to their rules, regulations and *modus operandi*, however illogical and condescending, and accept their service standards, no matter how shambolic. Just a few examples to illustrate the point.

- *Sitting in glorious sunshine at Taunton after a short rain delay, while the authorities debate whether it is permissible to use the light or heavy roller before play recommences, only for the matter to be then referred to Lord's HQ for prolonged arbitration.*
- *Arriving when the gates open at Southampton with a view to pre-match lunch, only to be told that because play commences at 2 p.m. and lunch is always two hours after the start of play, no food will be served until the luncheon interval at 4 p.m.*

- *Attending a Test match at Southampton on the promise of access to a private members' bar. The bar was there and fully stocked, but the door was locked throughout because of inexplicable ECB (England and Wales Cricket Board) regulations.*
- *Finding that it was not possible to buy a beer from the beer tent during a county match at Newport on the Isle of Wight because the barrel had run out and the next one would take two hours to settle. The alternative of a refreshing cup of tea was also temporarily off the menu because the urn was empty and would therefore need to be refilled and brought to the boil.*
- *A Test match ground running short of supplies on the second of five days because it had underestimated demand. They also failed to note that Christmas Day was on 25 December that year.*
- *Rules and regulations far too numerous to mention dictating what classes of ticket holder can access which seats and facilities at different times and under different conditions. Failure to adhere to these often unwritten or poorly communicated rules can lead to various sanctions, ranging from summary eviction to being barked at by Sergeant Major Square-Bash in a highly public and humiliating manner.*

The drinking cadre is not alone in offering the average patron a fascinating insight into the heterogeneity of human nature and the ability of groups and individuals to irritate and entertain in equal measure. Here are some of the thoughts and experiences I have gathered over the years.

- *The propensity of some to attend in fancy dress, and then behave in a manner incompatible with their adopted characters of nuns, monks, storm troopers and cartoon characters et cetera, accompanied by a bizarre fascination with the creation of "beer snakes" from empty beer containers. The semblance of brotherly love and bonding (they are usually always men!) gradually deteriorates during the day as evidenced one year at Southampton by a group of Fisherman's Friend lookalikes dressed in sou'westers, and their prey – a lobster. On leaving the ground, we discovered the lobster, having been chased around the stands all day by the sou'westers, abandoned in the gutter, cooked to a bright red hue!*
- *Colonel Cirrhosis creating a scene at Lord's, having been denied a double brandy at 10 a.m. He complained noisily and forcefully that he would not have been refused at any of his many other clubs across the UK!*
- *The foresight of those individuals who, over the years, have perfected the art of self-isolation by finding a seat in a completely empty stand, and managing to move to a similar situation should anyone dare to invade their enormous personal space.*
- *Hooray Henry from Hickstead accidentally slipping a foot into a tented makeshift latrine at Horsham and reacting by shouting, "Oops! Four faults!"*

So, it is not only in anticipation of a good day's play but also in the hope of some entertaining people-watching that we set off to various grounds.

We follow the fortunes of two teams. I have grown up being a Somerset supporter, as my mother hails from Taunton; likewise Vinny, who was brought up in Bath. However, we live in Hampshire and due to the ease with which we can get to the ground, plus Leah's brief county connection when performing as a Hampshire North wicketkeeper/batsman, we are members of Hampshire County Cricket Club. Consequently, we happily want both teams to win their matches – until crunch time when they play each other, in which case it is Somerset all the way.

Following cricket, like rugby, also provides good opportunities for travel and exploration. In 2017 we decided to do a tour of England, watching T20 cricket. We went from Kent, through Sussex and Hampshire, and on up through Nottinghamshire and Yorkshire to County Durham, before coming back down through Derbyshire, Leicestershire and Northamptonshire, with the sun setting on our tour back at the Ageas Bowl in Southampton.

In between games we visited a plethora of National Trust, English Heritage and privately owned properties, along with RHS gardens. We had weeks of glorious sunshine and a thoroughly enjoyable time in the English countryside.

The following year, our T20 tour started in Cheltenham, Gloucestershire, and carried on through the Cotswolds into Worcestershire, travelling back through the Wye Valley, the Forest of Dean, Chepstow down to Taunton, Somerset and back to Hampshire.

The summer of 2019 saw England and Wales hosting the Cricket World Cup. At Bristol for the Afghanistan versus Australia match, we realised that the relative cheers and boos given to the announcement of team members indicated that the crowd was very partisan towards Afghanistan, given who they were playing. At Taunton we once again watched Afghanistan bravely take on New Zealand.

At other matches, we witnessed the passions of the Indian supporters, who treated the event as a whole family day out; the depression of the West Indies supporters in the pouring rain; and the unbridled joy of the Bangladeshi supporters, who continually wound up the stewards by failing to remain in their allocated seats.

The semi-final at Edgbaston was on another level altogether. England blew the Aussies away. The atmosphere was electric, the crowd lustily singing "Cricket's Coming Home".

Only Vinny had been lucky enough to secure a ticket for the final at Lord's. I had to watch at home, Norma No Friends. But what a close and stunning win for England against New Zealand.

Over the years we have had many a trip to Lord's – Vinny being a member of the MCC – not just for T20 games but also for one-day matches, county games and Test matches.

During the latter I particularly recall gatherings on the lawn in the Coronation Garden during lunch breaks. It was quite fashionable, and still is to a limited extent, to lay down picnic blankets, before the start of play, round which friends would gather to share food and drink at lunchtime. It invariably became quite crowded and, at times of rain or on-field tedium, the risk of the conviviality extending well beyond the appointed break time was quite high.

As a source of tickets, Vinny was one of the organisers of such gatherings and attracted an eclectic but entertaining group with a hard core of regulars. (One of them was then a city financier and former concert pianist from Arkansas, who has since rediscovered God and is doing a splendid job preaching sermons in Scottish prisons while living in Ealing!)

A fellow organiser was the incomparable Gus who, as reported earlier, had once caused two nuns on a train enormous consternation by executing an irritant wasp and offering the consolation that he was now in 'the bosom of Abraham'. He usually held court (or attempted to) in a classic Falstaffian manner.

Although the group's hard core was very male-dominated, I was regarded as an honorary bloke, largely, I think, because I could hold my own in any sport-related conversation.

On one occasion, one of the regular members arrived with his cricket-loathing wife unexpectedly in tow. On being introduced, Falstaff bellowed to said friend with wife alongside, "My dear friend, I am sure we all have beautiful wives but that does not give us the liberty to inflict them on each other!" As always, he got away with the comment through his inimitable style of delivery which ensured that no-one, target included, could feel offended by what was said.

Our cricket lunches have not just been limited to these shores. We once partook of Christmas Day lunch in the pavilion at the Melbourne Cricket Ground in 2013 when the temperature outside was 40°C. We had travelled to Australia for the Fourth and Fifth Tests of that winter's Ashes tour.

We said beforehand that the worst-case scenario would be for England to be 3-0 down in the five-match series before we travelled out – and that, of course, is exactly what happened . .

. they lost the series 5-0! But we had a great time touring with Gullivers Travels, who basically provided the logistics and left clients free to engage in as much or as little group activity as they pleased. Leah has fond memories of a stunning New Year's Eve firework display over Sydney Harbour bridge viewed from a private launch in the close proximity of Port Jackson Bay. And of the week we spent near the Great Barrier Reef where she learned to scuba dive (while I took the easy option of walking down a ramp ten feet underwater wearing an air bell on my shoulders!)

As with rugby union in 2020, the cricket season was severely disrupted by Covid-19. The season was due to commence in April 2020, but it was not until July 2020 that the Government deemed it safe enough for, initially, Test match cricket to be played, albeit subject to certain caveats, including the exclusion of spectators. Cricket at county level was soon allowed to follow suit under similar restrictions.

At grass-roots level, those who play for the sheer love of the game were also permitted to don their whites again after some familiar Government U-turns in the face of high-profile celebrity challenges to the fundamental inconsistencies inherent in its evolving approach to the resumption of recreational sport.

A very late start to the 2020 cricket season meant that international, county, one-day and T20 fixtures had to be significantly reduced in number and condensed into the remaining summer and early autumn fair-weather window in dramatically reshaped competitive formats. All while players, officials and administrators adhered to new, demanding bio-secure regulations.

For once, the cricket authorities, including the England and Wales Cricket Board (ECB), excelled themselves and the arrangements they put in place made for a memorable few months of cricket. It was just so sad that we could not attend any matches in person – the first time this has happened to Vinny in over forty years – and that we had to rely on television to obtain our usual summer fix.

It was good to see England fare well in all formats of the game, but devastating to see Somerset once again fall just short of winning an elusive county title. For the umpteenth time Somerset finished as runners-up in the newly formatted county championship – always the bridesmaid but never the bride, having never won the championship since they first competed in the competition in 1891. As for Hampshire, who last won the championship in 1973, it was best to simply draw a discreet veil over the 2020 season.

The positions were reversed in the 2021 season with Hampshire being the bridesmaid and Somerset's charge fizzling out like a damp squib. You never know – in 2022 one of our teams might strike it lucky!

Although my interest in rugby and cricket can be fairly described as passionate – even bordering on the obsessive – I do enjoy a wide range of other sports in varying degrees. What, in cricketing terms, might be described as extras – or sundries, if you happen to be an Australian.

These extras include football, which I first experienced as a spectator at international level at Wembley in February 1979 when England beat Northern Ireland 4-0 in the qualifiers for Euro 80. The terraces were packed and I was the only female within a wide radius. Each time England scored, I was thrown into the air like a rag doll by exuberant supporters who, nevertheless, continually apologised for their language.

It was an exhilarating first taste of live international football, but it very nearly ended in disaster. Walking back to the underground station I was almost crushed by a massive police horse. I managed to get away with just a few minor bruises!

But the incident reminds me of a story a former police officer told me recently. Evidently, a female colleague was on crowd-control duty outside Stamford Bridge after a big Chelsea game. A passing drunken yob shouted up at her, "Oi, constable, your horse looks knackered!" To which she retorted, "So would you be if you had been between my legs for four hours!"

Another happy hunting ground has been Anfield, the home of Liverpool FC. I first went there in 1996 for the European Championship finals game between the Czech Republic and Italy that ended in a surprise 2-1 victory for the Czechs. I have always followed Liverpool for the highly tenuous reason that my late first husband, Julian, adopted them in the Sixties because their striker, Roger Hunt, was rebellious enough to play with his socks rolled down and sleeves rolled up!

In more recent years I have been able to fulfil a lifelong ambition by going to Anfield to watch Liverpool play in the Premier League. It was such a fantastic experience that I have been back on two other occasions. There is something special about joining in with a rousing rendition of "You'll Never Walk Alone".

It only proved possible to attend these games by obtaining a hospitality package on each occasion. In addition to match tickets, programme, three-course lunch in the Boot Room, post-match tea and a tour of the Liverpool FC museum, the club provided an entertainer and a former player to offer his predictions. On two occasions the latter was Phil Neal, and on the third, Jimmy Case.

Vinny accompanied me each time, of course, as did Leah on the first two. On the third visit, my brother-in-law Peter came with us. He announced over lunch that he was actually a Manchester United supporter. You can imagine how well received that was! Never again!

One of our visits to Anfield coincided with Vinny's birthday. At the last minute, due to television scheduling, the match was brought forward to 12 noon on Saturday, meaning that we had to travel up on Friday night. The inclusive lunch in the Boot Room became breakfast but the fare did not change. It was a bit bizarre being served roast beef and Yorkshire pudding with wine at 9 a.m.!

Because of the short notice, the only accommodation we could find beforehand was in Runcorn. That evening Vinny, Leah and I had a meal in the only decent-looking hostelry in downtown Runcorn – a Wetherspoon's – to celebrate said birthday. The total cost of the celebratory meal, including drinks, was £19.

To make matters worse for Vinny, but to Leah's and my delight, Liverpool beat Arsenal 5-1 the following day, after being 4-0 up within sixteen minutes. As a latent Arsenal supporter, I do not think Vinny has ever forgotten that birthday weekend!

Although I have continued to follow the progress of Liverpool and the national team, my love for football began to wane with the growth of supporter violence in the Eighties. Added to this was the escalation of footballers' wages (and with it, ticket prices), the concept of celebrity status that turned some players into prima donnas, and the business-driven fear of losing that took priority over the risk-ridden quest to win that has turned the game into a rather formulaic, predictable spectacle. In my view.

It might seem an awkward sideways leap from association football to tennis. But tennis has also formed another large sporting extra in my life, ever since my mother decided, during Wimbledon fortnight in the Sixties and Seventies, that Roach, Tanner and Borg represented a better televisual education for me than Rag, Tag and Bobtail.

Having used the BBC to indoctrinate me gently into the finer points of the game, my mother started taking me to Wimbledon in 1971, aged eleven, to see the world's finest players at first-hand and experience the special atmosphere that the tournament generates each year.

At that time, provided we were in the queue by 9 a.m., we would be guaranteed a seat on Centre or No. 1 Court. By the time I last went with her in 1984, we had to be in the queue by 5 a.m. Now, of course, people queue for several days.

We saw some fabulous tennis matches. In my youth, you could gain easy access to the show courts without a ticket at the end of each day. I recall watching Newcombe and Roche in a veterans' doubles match on Centre Court. The court was packed to the gunwales because, even as veterans, they were still very talented and hugely popular.

Occasionally my father was able to join us. I remember watching a doubles match with him on No. 2 Court involving Jimmy Connors and Ilie Năstase. Daddy repeated his great

Năstase quote. When asked by the police why he had not reported the theft of his credit card some months earlier, the great Romanian former World number one explained that it was because the thief was spending less than his wife!

Every year from 2000 to 2018 Vinny and I were fortunate enough to obtain tickets for Wimbledon in the public ballot. In 2004 we were allocated tickets for the Ladies' Final. Unfortunately, the tournament that year coincided with my first altercation with cancer and I was forced to watch the match from my hospital bed. But friends were able to enjoy the experience for us.

Fate looked kindly on me, however, because the following year we were again allocated tickets for the Ladies' Final and were this time able to attend in person to see Venus Williams defeat Lindsay Davenport in three sets.

Other sporting extras I have attended over the years have included golf at Wentworth, where I swooned as Seve Ballesteros passed within two feet of me at the Suntory World Match Play tournament in the Eighties; horse racing at various UK locations, including a memorable day at Newbury when I won £120; show jumping at Olympia, when an injured horse was sadly, and harrowingly, put down in the ring; rowing at Henley, where Vinny was once asked to stand in and start a race; ice hockey in Washington DC when one of the Washington Capitals players and an opponent were both sent to the sin bin for fighting even before the game started; and supporting the Boston Red Sox baseball team at Fenway Park during our family sojourn across the USA in 2012 (mentioned in chapter 14).

It is difficult to leave the subject of sport without mentioning the enormous contribution that commentators have made to my overall enjoyment of events when television or radio have had to take precedence over attendance at a live event.

When a sports commentator gets his or her observations wrong, whether knowingly or otherwise, the results can be spectacular in terms of amusement value. There are, of course, the classics, such as in cricket, for example, "The batsman's Holding, the bowler's Willey . . ."; in athletics, ". . . and there goes Juantorena down the back straight, opening his legs and showing his class!"; and in snooker, "For those of you watching in black and white, the pink is next to the green." The examples are legion!

The amusement value inherent in the commentator's art soon turns to irritation, however, as soon as the pre- or post-match interview starts with their stock question, "How important is it?" As in, how important is it for you to (a) win the match, (b) get through to the final, (c) outscore your opponent or (d) stay conscious. I'm still waiting for the day when the interviewee replies, "Not important at all – I don't care whether I win or lose!"

In the immortal words of the late, great Formula 1 commentator, Murray Walker, please "now excuse me while I interrupt myself" by moving from one lifelong passion – sport – to another. Travel.

12
A Thirst for Globetrotting

Watching live sport has always provided a good excuse for travel, but it has rarely been the sole, or even predominant, reason for jumping into the car or boarding an aeroplane. I firmly believe in the old adage that travel broadens the mind, and both Vinny and I have sought to exploit every possible opportunity to expand our horizons through sampling the varied histories, cultures and cuisine that exist across the globe. Although we have travelled extensively in fulfilment of our respective business commitments, the vast majority of our travel over the years has been for leisure purposes.

I believe my love of travel was sparked by those early school trips that my progressive primary school headmaster arranged, beginning when I was just seven years old.

I have since been lucky enough to visit a total of fifty-seven countries across six of the world's seven continents (the exception being Antarctica). I had plans to make that sixty, while I was sixty, with a trip to Uzbekistan in August 2020 to travel the Silk Road, with its cities of Bukhara, Tashkent and Samarkand, steeped in the history of Tamerlane. That was to be followed by a Central American tour of Honduras, Guatemala, El Salvador, Nicaragua and Costa Rica in the spring of 2021.

Unfortunately, the perfect storm created by a combination of my cancer diagnosis, associated broken neck and the Covid-19 travel restrictions, completely decimated those plans. I still intend to succeed with my target but accept that I will have to review the timing and choice of destinations!

In looking back for the purpose of this chapter, I determined from the outset that I did not want to create a form of travelogue, detailing my reminiscences of over fifty years of exploration, both at home and abroad. Even I would become bored and fall asleep part way through such a trawl.

Instead, I wanted to reflect on those events and incidents that have occurred on my travels that stand out as challenging, unusual, bizarre, surreal, frightening, hilarious or a combination thereof. Travelling in 2019 and 2020 with undiagnosed cancer and a broken neck has obviously added to my fund of stories in those categories, but I am pleased and relieved to say that they do not dominate in terms of either number or distinguishing characteristics!

Starting with the continent of Africa, Leah's love of animals and zoo visits made it almost inevitable that she would one day be petitioning us to choose a safari for our main family holiday. In the event, that did not happen until 2012 when she was fourteen years old. I responded by setting her the task of doing some research before proposing the optimum location and timing. I contributed to the research by describing my own experiences on the first safari holiday I undertook in 1990, when I visited Kenya, Tanzania and the Seychelles with my late first husband, Julian.

As with an incident in Barcelona many years later, described in the next chapter, this holiday included a strange encounter with foreign police officers.

While in a group of about ten people on a rickety bus that was well past its use-by date, travelling from Aruba in Tanzania to the Kenyan border, the vehicle was stopped at a roadblock and boarded by a scruffy bunch of police officers with carbines slung over their shoulders. They were looking for foreign currency, which at the time it was illegal to carry in Tanzania. When they realised that the only currency any of us possessed were Kenyan shillings, albeit still illegal, they were no longer interested. Clearly, they had been looking to confiscate dollars or sterling to boost their doubtless meagre incomes.

Leah's research in 2012 resulted in the suggestion that we visit Zambia, Botswana and South Africa during the summer of 2013. How could we resist? We started in Zambia in July 2013 where, from the back gate of our hotel, we were able to walk down to the stunning Victoria Falls. I recall the cheeky monkeys coming into our room to steal the paper-wrapped sugar cubes. Relaxing with Vinny and Leah sipping sundowners while gazing over the mighty Zambezi River was a particularly civilised experience. The three of us took a helicopter ride over the river and the falls, known locally as *Mosi-oa-Tunya* or "the smoke that thunders".

On leaving Zambia we crossed a 400-metre-wide part of the river by pontoon ferry from Kazungula into Botswana at a point where Zambia, Botswana, Namibia and Zimbabwe meet. It's known as the "four corners of Africa", so we were very much in deepest Africa at this point.

In Botswana we stayed in a remote lodge run by a charming British couple in the Chobe National Park. During our stay we were lucky enough to see, at varying times of day and night, the "Big Five" comprising leopard, lion, buffalo, elephant and rhinoceros, as well as countless giraffe, impala, hyenas and vultures.

But as with a sunny day out at the cricket, people-watching was also rarely off our agenda. On one excursion, as we were gazing at some lionesses stalking zebra on the edge of the savannah, one of our party asked the guide, rather undiplomatically, which nationality sat at the top of the list of most annoying or irritating tourists. He said Americans, but with some hesitation given the presence of an elderly and inoffensive American couple within our number. He went on to explain that their most irritating trait, in his humble opinion, was to shout, "Oh my God" as often and loudly as they possibly could.

Just as he said that, and with great comedic timing, a small number of Land Cruisers pulled up nearby and offloaded their American cargo. As soon as their eyes had been guided to the wildlife populating the plains, they shouted "Oh my God" in perfect unison. Luckily, we were hidden from their view, so they could not see us contorted in laughter at their expense. As for the accompanying noise, we just hoped that they put it down to an unseen and unknown species.

From Chobe we flew down to the Okavango Delta on a nine-seater plane, landing on a small grass airstrip from where a boat took us and our luggage to our hotel, deep in the heart of the delta.

We ventured out on the delta each day on a *mokoro*, accompanied by one or two guides, to explore the flora and fauna, including the extensive variety of birdlife. It was glorious. Each day's adventure ended with gin or vodka and tonic in hand watching, in total silence from the rear of the *mokoro*, the sun setting fast over the delta.

On one such trip we moored the *mokoro* in a remote location and set out on foot – just the three of us and two local guides – for an exploration of the immediate vicinity. The unarmed guides provided us with no more than some rudimentary safety instructions. They explained that elephants have poor vision and operate more on scent than sight. Consequently, they do not charge at a potential threat without first doing a dummy run and stopping just short to see if the target moves. If it does move, the elephant will wander downwind to prepare for the real thing.

Having got too close and personal for comfort with some hippopotami (who kill more humans than elephants do each year), we unexpectedly encountered a lone bull elephant on turning a sharp corner. This elephant dutifully prepared to charge us. As instructed by our guides we grabbed hold of each other in a single line and remained absolutely still (not easy to do!!) as the elephant charged straight at us. Luckily, it was a mock-charge, and so the elephant stopped just short of us before slowly moving away.

I would not say I was petrified, but when the guide tapped me on the shoulder to say I could now move, I found I had become frozen to the spot with my forehead implanted in Leah's shoulder.

The rest of the walking tour was less than relaxing, and we voted for a swift return to base for a change of underwear and a stiff drink.

We spent our last evening on the delta having dinner with a charming Dutch family, before embarking the following day on our journey to Cape Town via Botswana's capital, Gaborone.

The flight to Gaborone took off from the same delta airstrip on which we had landed a few days beforehand. There was just a slight delay before departure as the young pilot used this transit stop to eat her sandwiches as we sat alongside her and chatted on the dried mud runway.

On arrival in Cape Town, the locals expressed surprise that we had left behind a British summer for a South African winter. But with blue skies and temperatures in the thirties in Zambia and Botswana, followed by more blue sky and a temperature of twenty degrees in Cape Town, we were more than happy.

I have an unenviable record for visiting cities with iconic sights at a time when such sights are inaccessible due to weather conditions or other acts of God. The Empire State Building in New York (fog) and Mount Fuji in Japan (low cloud) spring readily to mind. It therefore came as no surprise that at the time of our visit to Cape Town, the Table Mountain cable car was closed for a programme of maintenance that takes place every six years. Vinny suggested that we walk up to the top, but Leah and I were not so keen.

But this setback did not dampen our spirits and we saw as much of Cape Town on foot as we possibly could. Obviously, we had to be careful, and having on one occasion been told by a local to put my camera away, we decided to explore most districts from the safety of a vehicle.

We also took the opportunity to visit Robben Island, where our guide for the tour of the prison was a former fellow inmate of Nelson Mandela.

Naturally, we enjoyed wine-tasting in Stellenbosch and travelled down to the Cape itself. Normally one expects the wind and rain at the Cape to blow trees and humans into the horizontal position, particularly at the time of year we visited.

But we struck lucky in that the sun decided to shine from a cloudless sky.

It was while in Cape Town that Vinny reminded me of an interesting business trip that he had made to the African continent in the early Nineties. He accompanied the government's then immigration minister on a mad fact-finding trip to East and West Africa, covering seven countries in twelve days. Also on the trip was the minister's private secretary, Digby (his real name, so I do not have to invent an appropriate pseudonym!)

When in Nairobi, an afternoon's schedule of engagements was unexpectedly cancelled due to a local difficulty. To get the small party out of his hair, the high commissioner, with whom they were staying, loaned them his jeep and driver so that they could enjoy the wildlife in the Nairobi National Park.

With no time to change, they headed off into the deep heat of the afternoon, still dressed in their suits and ties. It got dark very early in Nairobi during the season of their visit and the gates to the park closed sharply at 6 p.m.

As a rather surreal afternoon drew to a close the jeep began to move at greater speed and the driver's skills became more reckless. When he reversed out of yet another cul-de-sac, with the eyes of a huge confusion of wildebeest glinting in the headlights, the following stilted exchange took place.

Vinny: "Are you sure, driver, you are familiar with all of the park's exit routes?"

Driver: "Oh yes, sir, yes, sir!"

Vinny: (glancing disbelievingly at the minister and Digby)

Minister: "Are you fully prepared, Digby, should we be locked in the park overnight?"

Digby: "Yes, minister. I took the precaution of placing an extra tube of Trebor Mints and a Swiss army knife in my briefcase."

Minister: "Good man, Digby. I knew I could rely on you at a time of crisis."

Silence then descended as the driver, more by luck than judgement, found the necessary escape route and raced through the exit gates at 5.57 p.m. At that moment there was just one final utterance.

Minister: "Now that we have escaped with our lives, Digby, I want you to search my room when we get back. I feel sure I have mislaid my comb!"

A fine example of British stoicism in the face of extreme danger post the dying embers of Empire!

Moving from Africa to the Americas, my first trip across the pond was to New York City in 1979. Back then it was a pretty scary place. It was not safe to travel on the subway and not much better on foot. I recall, while walking past a large residential building, a motorcyclist driving round the block in a continuous circuit. Suddenly, a man ran out waving a firearm, shouting, "If he comes again, I'll shoot him." Taxi!

We did not feel much safer when visiting Philadelphia, but such experiences were nicely balanced by a delightful drive up through New York State and across to the Canadian side of Niagara Falls.

I returned to New York in 2007 with Vinny and Leah for what proved to be a much more relaxing trip. The whole atmosphere was open and friendly, and we were able to get around without feeling in any way threatened or uncomfortable.

We took in all the major attractions, including a fog-shrouded Empire State Building, and secured tickets for *Chicago* on Broadway. We stayed just off Time Square, where we found a delightful deli for our morning bagels. As we entered on the third morning, the server was already preparing our order. The Americans certainly know how to do hospitality.

The strangest and most harrowing part of the short break had to be seeing Ground Zero, having been to the top of the Twin Towers on my first visit nearly thirty years previously.

My first visit to California in 1982, while on a road trip that also covered Arizona and Nevada, had resulted in another entertaining encounter with a foreign police officer. We stopped in Carmel-by-Sea, Clint Eastwood's home town. Initially we parked on the edge of town.

The combination of huge roadside parking bays and a small hire car meant we inadvertently parked across two bays. We returned to a parking violation notice on the windscreen.

Later we moved to the main drag. Unfortunately, that invoked another parking violation, this time for parking more than two metres from the kerb. The car was parked facing the wrong way! Muttering, "This is ridiculous!", we stomped in high dudgeon into the local sheriff's office to complain.

Sheriff Two Ton emerged, complete with regulation shades, pistols and chewing gum. Wind rapidly left our sails. "You English, why y'all complain about your parking tickets?" In a nod to transatlantic relations, he ripped one up and handed the other back with a stern warning to pay it before leaving the country. We left his office with tail between legs, despite the minor victory!

That road trip also included a visit to the Grand Canyon with a flight on a four-seater Cessna flown by a Dutch pilot who did her training at Blackbushe Airfield, not far from where we now live in Hampshire. The ninety-minute duration of the flight meant that we were able to travel a long distance and beyond the range of other sightseeing aircraft. This led our pilot to break the regulations by flying down below the lip of the canyon itself.

We returned to the West Coast in May 2008, having accepted, in a moment of sheer impulse, a verbal invitation from a barrister friend to attend her Hindu wedding at Huntingdon Beach, California.

Not only did we happily sign up to attend, but I also agreed to Anita's suggestion that I should wear a *shalwar kameez*. She took me to all the best Indian couturiers in Wembley High Street, London. I chose some ivory silk with brocade and also chiffon from which the outfit was handmade. Gorgeous but understated!

Once I was back home, after being told the cost, Vinny commented in his usual measured way, "We could have flown to California first class for that price but I do, of course, respect your choice!" I, in return, respected the choice of both Vinny and Leah to dress a tad more conservatively!

I was very anxious that wearing a traditional outfit should not cause any cultural offence. This was particularly so, given that we were one of only three white families who had travelled to attend the wedding. But, of course, Anita was absolutely right.

I received so many wonderful compliments – plus gratitude for choosing to wear the outfit. It hangs in my wardrobe thirteen years on, still waiting for the next suitable occasion!

While staying at Huntingdon Beach, we naturally visited Beverly Hills and Hollywood, including Sunset Strip and Hollywood Boulevard with its walk of fame. We also visited Universal Studios where, as in much of the USA, *Elf and Safety* do not really feature.

On the tour of the lots, we witnessed King Kong hanging off a burning skyscraper, drove through the parting of the Red Sea, and saw a burning plane heading towards us before crashing into a lake, as per a scene from Kevin Costner's *Waterworld*. Everywhere we walked there were collapsing buildings, machine-gun fire and genuine flames.

At the studios we went on one of the best rides we have ever experienced – *The Simpsons*. It was a virtual roller coaster. We were strapped into seats in a pitch-black studio while surrounded by an animated ride on a huge screen. The seats jolted and moved on their bases, creating the very real physical sensation that you were actually on the ride. I normally hate roller coasters but this was brilliant. If there had not been a long queue, we would have been straight back on it. Looking back, it all makes sense now that I know the difference between *basophobia* and *acrophobia*!

We also visited nearby Disneyland, where we went on another fantastic ride – *Star Wars*. It operated according to the same principle as *The Simpsons* ride, but this time creating the sensation of making a hyper-leap through space while under attack from Empire star destroyers. The queue was very long, but the likes of C-3PO and R2-D2 helped the time slip past by providing entertainment along the line.

The main purpose of our visit, the wedding itself, took place in the grounds of our hotel in Huntingdon Beach. The groom, who had variously been involved in the fields of law, neurosurgery and finance, arrived on an elephant. A somewhat incongruous sight on the streets of Orange County suburbia adjacent to the Atlantic! But a truly outstanding experience nonetheless.

South America is much less familiar to me than North America, but one trip there does stand out by virtue of a stunning visit we made to Ecuador for a stay in Quito, followed by a cruise around the Galápagos Islands.

Out of the blue my mother announced in 2007 that she would like Vinny and I to take her to the Galápagos Islands for her eightieth birthday. Right oh, Mother, as you do!

So in February 2008, Vinny and I, accompanied by Leah and Granny, set off to celebrate the latter's big Eight O, somewhat prematurely, having booked a package (the only viable option) through *Voyages Jules Verne*. We joined a small group of fourteen fellow travellers at Heathrow Airport. Although the rest of the group were mainly retired, they proved good, lively companions, united by a keen interest in travel generally, but the unique flora and fauna of the Galápagos in particular.

We flew Iberia to Quito via Madrid where the fun began. Although we had obviously been through security at Heathrow, and remained airside on arrival at Madrid, the chaotic Spanish authorities insisted that all passengers go through security again. The only problem was that the early shift had not yet arrived to open the security gate.

Pandemonium ensued as all the passengers trapped on the wrong side of the locked gate were connecting with flights for various South American cities, and many of those flights had already been called.

We eventually navigated this unnecessary pinch point when staff arrived with minutes to spare, only to discover that our flight, which was closing, was departing from the furthest gate possible. Vinny and Leah ran ahead to hold the fort while I ushered Granny and the slower members of the group. We all made it on to the plane to a round of applause from the waiting passengers already on board.

After a few nights in Quito, we flew to the Galápagos. Transfer from the airport to the boat, which accommodated about 100 passengers, was by RIB. Once alongside our cruise boat, we were advised to slide alternately down the side walls of the RIB, where we had been seated, then step on to the ladder for the boat. What did Granny do? Stand up and walk down the centre of the RIB. What happened? She fell in a heap!

On board all passengers were divided into teams for the purposes of visiting individual islands. Thanks to the near military-like organisational skills of the crew and the Galápagos National Park, the teams did not mingle when exploring the islands, and we rarely encountered groups from other boats. Our team was named the Blue-footed Boobies, which we considered appropriate given that family Hogg wore bright blue Crocs throughout the trip – a statement of sartorial elegance that I am not sure Leah fully appreciated.

Only four of the islands are inhabited, the main ones being Santa Cruz and San Cristobal. The Charles Darwin centre is located on San Cristobal, where we immersed ourselves in a long and fascinating ecology lesson before embarking on a walking tour of the local sights. These included the small harbourside fish market, with its swarm of hungry pelicans creating a scene reminiscent of the animated film, *Finding Nemo*.

But the majority of islands we visited were uninhabited, apart from the stunning variety of wildlife, including the ubiquitous iguana, which had become accustomed to human visitors getting up close and personal without posing a threat.

The flora and scenery were equally breathtaking, while Leah was able to enjoy several swimming and snorkelling excursions among the amazing marine life. We felt so privileged to have been allowed to step into this special world where so much is done to protect the exceptional habitat while still allowing a limited, but financially vital, amount of tourism.

At the time of our visit, Lonesome George, the famous Pinta Cruz giant tortoise, was still alive and captivated us all. Leah did an exceptional presentation on him on her return to school. Sadly, George died in 2012, aged in excess of 100, having failed to father a single hatchling during his lifetime.

Granny managed to get through the week, climbing in and out of the RIB for our daily island visits, with just one other fall. This occurred when she was exiting on to a jetty, but it did not deter her. Some years later she did comment that if she had not travelled to the Galápagos when she did, she would never have been fit enough to do so. It really was a trip of a lifetime, and we felt indebted to my mother for suggesting such a novel way to celebrate her eightieth birthday – and directing that we take her!

My previous trip to South America had been in 1992 to Rio de Janeiro for the *Mardi Gras* carnival. The memory of sitting on the stone steps of the Sambadrome at 3 a.m. in temperatures of thirty degrees, while watching 5,000 dancers samba past, is etched on my mind.

A slightly more eccentric episode involved a tour of the great Maracanã Stadium (sadly left to rack and ruin after the 2016 Olympics), led by an aged Portuguese-only-speaking boot boy, that culminated in taking a seat in the dugout looking out over the pitch.

In many ways these two contrasting memories sum up the overall impression I was left with on returning home after two weeks in Brazil. Namely, that the citizens appeared either extremely rich or mired in abject poverty, with very little grey colouring in between. But everybody we met appeared to be happy and fun-loving, regardless of which side of the social divide they sat.

The same could be said of the people we met in India, where Vinny and I went for a tour of the Golden Triangle in 2012 for his sixtieth birthday.

Again, we chose *Voyages Jules Verne*, given the complications of individually tailored travel to that part of the world. We joined a small group of around twelve people, and we all got on well.

On arrival in Jaipur, where we were staying at the Maharajah's Palace, our tour guide mentioned that one couple might be lucky enough to be allocated the maharajah's suite.

At this point Vinny decided to have a quiet word with the tour manager. Using a degree of reverse psychology, he argued that any decision on allocation must be done on a fair and equal basis, and no account should be taken of the fact that it was his, Vinny's, sixtieth birthday. We were given the keys to the suite.

The maharajah's suite was mightily impressive. We entered via the anteroom, twice the size of our sitting room. From there we moved through the ballroom, half the size of a football pitch, to our exceedingly spacious bedroom, dressing room and bathroom. We even had our own private garden. Later we were told that Prince Charles had stayed in the suite with both Diana and Camilla, although it was never made clear whether that was on the same or different occasions!

Like Princess Diana, Vinny was later photographed at the Taj Mahal but he was unable to attract the same level of attention, despite it being the day he turned sixty.

Given the amount of travelling that we have been lucky enough to undertake, the law of averages dictates that not everything will go according to plan all of the time. I have already mentioned the Empire State Building being shrouded in fog (as the tour guide said incredulously as we entered the lift, "You guys are crazy – there is zero visibility up there!"); Mount Fuji covered by low cloud; and Table Mountain rendered inaccessible by cable-car maintenance.

The family holiday in Barbados in January 2005 presented our longest run of disappointments over the course of a single two-week vacation. This was intended to be a replacement holiday for the planned 2004 summer alpine trip to Lake Bled, Slovenia, which we had to cancel due to my first cancer diagnosis. (Actually, that turned out to be a stroke of good fortune. We recently had a long weekend in Ljubljana, and a day trip to Lake Bled left us wondering what, if we had visited in 2004, we would have done on the other thirteen days!)

We chose this time of year because it is the height of the

Caribbean holiday season, with wall-to-wall sunshine almost guaranteed. The island is only twenty-one by fourteen miles and there is not a lot to do there if you are not interested in watersports.

The only real attraction is the spectacular Harrison Cave. Unfortunately, it teemed with rain the whole time we were on Barbados. The cave was flooded and closed!

But the *pièce de résistance* has to be our trip to Malta in 2017. The must-see UNESCO world heritage site, Ħal Saflieni Hypogeum, was closed for essential maintenance and the Azure Window, a natural limestone arch formed in the nineteenth century, which was the major attraction on the island of Gozo and has featured in a number of international films and media productions, collapsed into the sea a few days before we arrived!

We mentioned some of these disappearing or invisible must-sees and other incidents to our fellow Rugby World Cup travellers, in the context of the cancelled England versus France game, while involved in the aforementioned pub quiz on the forty-fifth floor of our Tokyo hotel as Typhoon Hagibis raged outside in 2019.

The response was that if they had known our track record beforehand, they would have booked a different trip. The moral of the story is, if you want to see the top sights in the world, do not travel with the Hoggs!

Naturally, much of our overseas travel has involved flying, a subject worthy of mention in itself. There are almost inevitably the occasional cancellations and extreme delays. I have previously mentioned being marooned by Storm Clara in Nice and Typhoon Hagibis in Tokyo. While on business in Bermuda, Vinny had perhaps a more unusual reason for a delayed flight and a stay extended by a couple of days – celebrations on the runway to mark National Day!

There are the more common, but potentially alarming experiences. White-knuckle descents into Belfast because of crosswinds. Amazing reflections of planes on skyscrapers while descending into Kai Tak, Hong Kong. Multiple attempts to land at Funchal, Madeira.

Then there are the one-offs, the unexpected. Domestic flights in China provide fertile ground here. On descending into Xian on a China Northwest Airlines flight from Beijing, the pilot came in far too quickly. He landed with a hefty thump and slammed on the anchors. I was bodily thrown into the back of the seat in front of me. I apologised to the woman seated there but was reassured by her that I had not caused her any discomfort as she had been similarly attached to the seat in front of her.

The arrival at Guilin on a China Southwest Airlines flight from Shanghai was equally dramatic. We touched down only seconds after emerging from thick cloud. The next morning the clear weather allowed us to appreciate the sheer beauty of Guilin but I was horrified to discover we were surrounded by mountains. Apparently, we should not have landed but we were unable to return to Shanghai because it was snowbound.

Vinny's solo experiences include a descent into Lagos on a Nigerian Airlines flight similar to the full-throttle approach in Xian. All of the ill-fitting and mismatched seats, which appeared to have been sourced from a local breaker's yard, shook violently, and he could see the looks of horror on the faces of the crew through the badly stained and torn dividing curtain!

On boarding a PIA flight somewhere in Asia many years ago, he was horrified to see fellow travellers cooking their breakfast on a primus stove in the aisle.

The announcements can be equally worrying. On a Balkan Air flight to Sofia the silence was broken by an announcement that went, "Emergency, Emergency. Please listen very carefully. We have no hot water and cannot, therefore, serve tea or coffee."

On an internal flight in the US the captain suddenly announced, as we approached Chicago, "This is a message for passenger X –" (name publicly announced) – "We have just heard from the Alabama Corrections Department that it will now be possible for you to deplane at O'Hare without fear of arrest." And, of course, I have already mentioned how the Bath Rugby team supposedly compromised weight distribution on the descent into Claremont.

On our travels around the world I have, for some unknown reason, developed a mild obsession for visiting Hard Rock Cafes whenever the opportunity arises. Some of them are fairly centrally located and easy to find, such as in San Francisco, Memphis, Seattle and New Orleans. Others are, or were, further out of the city centre, as in Sydney. Even in London, the original is situated a little out of the way at the far end of Piccadilly. It is not always easy to find them, requiring a special trip diverting us from normal city sightseeing!

It is the merchandise and rock memorabilia that attracts me rather than the culinary fare. I now have a great selection of T-shirts. Sadly, I did not have the foresight when I purchased them to check whether the neckline was large enough to go over a neck brace.

However, the menu did have its uses while in Japan, given my seafood allergy. So, finding Hard Rock Cafes in Tokyo and Kyoto was a real bonus on the epicurean front (even our fellow travellers asked us for directions).

Locating the Kyoto café was a real challenge. Not only was it tucked away, but it looked the least like a Hard Rock Cafe as one could imagine. From the outside it could easily have been mistaken for a traditional Japanese tea garden. Inside was just like a Japanese restaurant with accompanying customs – a most interesting experience.

Drawing on these recollections of some wonderful travels across the globe proved really uplifting as I simultaneously began to contemplate a much narrower set of options for future adventures. It also served to demonstrate how happy memories can improve a positive state of mind, and underlined the importance of not deferring to a far-off date those must-dos or must-sees on one's bucket list! Luckily, I have always resisted the temptation to do that, preferring instead to turn my travel dreams into early fulfilment.

13

Travel Closer to Home

I have already touched upon the fact that Vinny and I have both travelled quite extensively for business purposes. Vinny spent a fair proportion of his time travelling overseas, particularly in the Nineties and Noughties. Like many frequent flyers he had two passports so that he could travel on one while applying for visas for future planned trips with the other. When not abroad, he was often overnighting across the UK.

When he was at home, my duty solicitor commitments frequently meant that I was called out in the evening, in the middle of the night and at weekends. On top of that my military work often entailed me travelling abroad, particularly to Germany but also beyond. Luckily, as you will have appreciated, our shared leisure interests meant that we were able to maximise our downtime together in pursuit of joint distractions.

If the opportunity arose, I would try and accompany Vinny on visits (at our own expense, of course), but such occasions proved to be rare. Indeed, I can count them on barely two hands – Barcelona, Dublin, Vienna (twice), Sofia and, UK-wise, York. But each one, nevertheless, evokes vivid memories.

Barcelona is a wonderful city with a warm atmosphere that can be felt as soon as one steps out on to the streets – a city that definitely benefits from pedestrian exploration. *Las Ramblas*, the *Sagrada Familia* and the Gaudi architecture are must-views. I have been there a number of times but while visiting in the early Noughties, when Vinny chaired a European policing conference in the city, we were involved in a most entertaining encounter.

It was half term, so I paid for Leah and myself to go out and join him, do some child-friendly sightseeing and then spend a family weekend together.

At the start of the weekend, we were on our way to *Plaça de Catalunya* when suddenly a police car screeched up beside us and out jumped, *Oficial* Cocky and *Oficial* Obnoxious both clad in shades while chewing gum. Cocky was the gobby one while Obnoxious smirked inanely doing his back-up job. The exchange went as follows.

> *Oficial Cocky: (invading personal space and being extremely aggressive) "Passports, now!"*
> *Vinny: (smiling pleasantly, hands over passports)*
> *Oficial Cocky: "What are you doing?"*
> *Vinny: "We're on our way to* Plaça de Catalunya."
> *Oficial Cocky: (still very aggressive) "Where have you been?"*
> *Vinny: "I've just been chairing a conference attended by your boss, the Chief of Catalonian Police."*
> *Oficial Cocky: (turning white in the face and stepping back) "Ah, ah, we've had reports of a Russian family illegally changing money on the street."*
> *Vinny: "Do we look like Russian money-changers?"*
> *Oficial Cocky: "No, no, no. Have a nice day." (handing passports back)*

Cocky and Obnoxious could not get back in their car quickly enough.

Dealing with foreign police officers can be entertaining as this and my earlier stories hopefully illustrate!

For the trip to Dublin, I naturally flew on a commercial flight, unlike Vinny, who had earlier accompanied the then PM, Tony Blair, on the UK's equivalent of Air Force One from Northolt.

I recall my taxi ride from the airport – the driver emitted a constant stream of disconnected verbiage. It reminded me of my father's favourite comment about my mother – "I'm afraid my wife has a speech impediment; she has to stop talking in order to draw breath!"

While in Dublin for the weekend we took in all the tourist sites (it was my first visit there), as well as some of the *craic* and the Guinness (of course!). A wonderful city to which we have returned a number of times.

For several years Vinny led the UK delegation at an annual UN drugs policy conference in Vienna. I was able to join him on two occasions, once with Leah and once without.

Leah fared well out of these trips, even when not travelling with me, although she did not appreciate this at the time. Vinny bought her a Steiff bear but, of course, she was never allowed to play with it. Twenty years on it remains in pristine condition and she has come to cherish it.

I, on the other hand, bought her a wonderful animal-print outfit that, fortunately, she got much wear out of. At the time I managed to misread the decimal point in the purchase price. I turned pale when Vinny gently pointed out that there is a big difference between €30 and €300!

Vienna was unlucky for me in another way in that I had a

whole pint tipped over my coat in a bar. Some Austrians can be rather brusque at times, and I was made to feel it was my fault. But overall, two very enjoyable trips with plenty of sightseeing while Vinny was working.

The visit to Sofia was most enlightening. I was met at the airport and whisked into the city for afternoon tea with Vinny and his colleague then stationed in Bulgaria.

That evening we went to not one, but *three* embassy receptions – parties, in other words! At one, I met people who had been on a posting in Islamabad with the parents of a school friend of Leah. It's a small world.

Although an enjoyable evening, I felt as though I was effectively "on duty". But I did make up for it with a weekend of interesting events, including a standing-room-only classical concert in a vast, dusty church, and a visit to a Russian restaurant clearly run by the local mafia!

I cannot say that I altogether miss the days when Vinny was forever packing or unpacking suitcases, and taking a taxi to Heathrow on a Sunday afternoon while I was stuck in a police station in Aldershot or Basingstoke or heading to the airport for regular overseas military cases. But our respective consultancy years, with my more measured approach and Vinny's switch to just occasional visits to the likes of Paris, Brussels, Tbilisi, Yerevan and Istanbul have provided a useful transition from manic globetrotting to Covid-19 lockdown. Not that we knew what was in store for 2020 at the time!

European city breaks for leisure purposes have always been high on the wish list. I much prefer to visit a city on foot, if possible, to take in the sights and smells, but sometimes one has to avail oneself of public transport in the larger cities, and thinking of that brings to mind a long weekend we spent with Swedish friends, Hans and Siw, at their home in Stockholm during the 2002 Football World Cup hosted by Japan. Vinny met Hans during a number of international business trips around twenty-five years ago and our families have remained firm friends ever since.

It just so happened that during our stay England played Sweden in the group stage of the World Cup. We therefore settled down at their home to watch the game on television. Hans and Siw had bravely bucked the trend in their street by flying both the Swedish flag and the Union Jack outside their home.

Clearly aware of our situation, and to assist diplomatic harmony, the England team contrived to concede an equaliser through a Danny Mills second-half blunder and so the game finished 1-1. What relief – a close friendship protected!

The England goal was scored by Sol Campbell, which sparked a conversation between us about the meaning of the word *Sol*. On hearing my pathetic utterance that I thought *Sol* was the French word for *sun*, Leah, who had been sitting quietly in the corner, contemplating her fifth birthday the following day, suddenly exclaimed, "No, Mummy, the word is *soleil*!" Hans and Siw have never forgotten that moment!

Hans and Siw kindly took us on a magnificent tour of their familiar haunts, including their lovely remote family summer home, a visit to Uppsala, and the main attractions of

Stockholm. The latter included the *Vasa* Museum, where Leah chose a rat as her soft toy gift!

It really was the most perfect weekend, blessed by great company and warm summer sun.

On leaving the centre of Stockholm one afternoon, we travelled on an extremely busy metro train with a very tired Leah sitting on my lap. Unfortunately, her foot skimmed against the woman opposite, who scowled at me and brushed her suit trouser leg in a manner that played to the gallery. Shortly thereafter the seat next to me became available and I very carefully lifted Leah into it. As I did so, her foot again accidentally touched the woman's leg. This time she dusted her leg down in very dramatic style and, in English, had a right go at me for not keeping my child under control.

Before I had a chance to respond, numerous passengers around us stepped in and loudly rebuked her – also in English – so that we could understand, about her behaviour towards English guests and an innocent child. She got off at the next stop.

We found the Swedish welcome and hospitality absolutely stunning and never to be forgotten. As an aside, we were able to return some British hospitality when Hans and Siw came over to stay with us for my fiftieth birthday celebrations, held in a marquee in our garden.

The following morning, Jo opened the village shop specially to provide them (and us) with an excellent full English breakfast. Such happy times.

I have already mentioned visiting Paris on a number of occasions, including to watch Bath play *Stade Français* in the semi-final of the European Challenge Cup in 2017.

Another reason to travel there was for a four-day visit to Disneyland Paris in 2001 for Leah's fourth birthday. My mother came with us.

In those days, Eurostar operated out of Waterloo, so catching the Disney Express direct from Waterloo International to Disneyland Paris could not have been easier for residents of north-east Hampshire. On checking in at Waterloo, we were issued with our four-day passes.

On arrival at Disneyland Paris, we were able to go straight into the park while our luggage was delivered to the hotel. I will never forget the look on Leah's face as we were immediately greeted by a huge Mickey Mouse – and similar excitement when we later bumped into Pooh Bear.

There were so many magical rides and attractions suitable for a four-year-old and, I have to admit, three rather wimpish adults. My mother's favourite was *It's a Small World*, a boat ride through various areas of the world, featuring audio-animatronic dolls in traditional costume, singing the attraction's title song.

The four of us were also able to fit into one of the Mad Hatter's teacups on his unbirthday whirligig, which Leah enjoyed spinning around. She also insisted that we watch the grand parade each afternoon, principally, I suspect, to see the fire- and smoke-breathing dragon with its various wires inadvertently hanging out of its mouth. But Leah was not best pleased with Vinny on the rope-bridge for deliberately making it wobble and causing her granny consternation. Leah had to put on her best caring head and help Granny across.

One evening, Vinny and I went back into the park to experience some of the more adventurous rides while Granny stayed at the hotel with Leah. Unfortunately, one of Leah's then favourite toys – Skinny, a long-legged mouse – slipped down between the beds and got left behind. Granny was mortified and never forgot it (although she may have done so now that dementia has set in!).

On the day of Leah's fourth birthday, the lights suddenly dimmed during dinner and she was thrilled to see the waiting staff come in singing 'Happy Birthday' and carrying a huge cake bedecked with candles. Seconds later, she was crestfallen as they went to another table. A few minutes later, though, the same process happened again and this time they came to our table. Although the element of surprise was gone, she was still delighted.

The cake was too large for us, so we sliced up the remainder and Leah took it round to children on other tables.

As we left the park on the last day, Leah had to let her Minnie Mouse helium balloon go, as it could not come back on the train with us. But we all smiled as we watched it sail away because it had been such a magical few days. Like some parents who take their children to Disneyland, I doubt very much that we admitted looking forward to the visit beforehand!

A dual-city break back in 2000 involved Vinny and I visiting Prague and Budapest, with a train ride connecting the two. Both cities were a delight to visit, but two amusing incidents jump to mind.

We were on a *Voyages Jules Verne* trip where the party numbered ten. As we were on a group ticket for the train journey, one of us had to be appointed lead traveller. The VJV rep, who was not taking the train with us, handed this role to one who could only be described as Captain Mainwaring the Second. Once on the train, he allocated us seats with another couple in one carriage while he and his new chums took the seats in a second carriage. He believed he was punishing us for refusing to admire his pomposity during our time in Prague. However, it suited us as we promptly took ourselves off to the bar, nabbed seats facing a full window and had a thoroughly enjoyable three-hour journey taking in the stunning scenery, along with a libation or two!

Whilst in Budapest, we booked dinner at a smart restaurant with a fine reputation, where access was gained through an upmarket antique shop. The meal was exquisite with excellent blinis, caviar and champagne for starters. Unfortunately, it was all spoiled when it came to payment. Before attending, we had checked that Visa was acceptable and this was confirmed by the presence of the Visa logo on the door of the restaurant. On presentation of our card the waiters demanded cash – florints at the time. There was a long stand-off during which we resolved that washing-up was definitely not going to be a possible route out. We could have part-paid using the florints we had brought with us for an intended tip, but determined not to on a point of principle.

We eventually won the day, and they lost out on the handsome tip we would have left for what, up until that point, had been an exemplary meal and service.

As previously mentioned we visited Berlin in October 2003 where we stayed at The Hotel Adlon. It has, over the years, had many famous celebrity guests, including, from the Golden Twenties, the likes of Charlie Chaplin and Marlene Dietrich.

In modern times, Michael Jackson is remembered for dangling his infant son, Prince Michael II ("Blanket"), out of the window. Leah Hogg is less well remembered for spending time in the corridor swapping all the shoes that had been placed outside bedroom doors for cleaning.

Our trip to Berlin was the first holiday that we had arranged ourselves, rather than through an agent, by booking both flights and hotel online. We had originally sourced the trip through a holiday company but I decided to check relative costs on the internet. To my astonishment, by booking flights and the hotel direct, we could save £750. We have never looked back. Mind you, it was just as well, given that breakfast for the four of us for four nights came to £350!

A European multi-city break with a difference saw us visit all three capitals of the Baltic States, travelling by private taxi between Vilnius in Lithuania, Riga in Latvia and Tallinn in Estonia, before concluding our trip in Copenhagen, Denmark.

In each of the Baltic capitals we had a day or half-day walking tour with a local, personal guide. It proved an excellent way to learn about the history and culture of each of the three countries, although we felt suitably chastised by our local guide in Vilnius – on behalf of all Western European visitors – for taking such an unhealthy interest in the KGB museum.

The only drawback to the trip was the decision to fly Ryanair from Luton – an experience that I would not wish to repeat in a hurry. Returning alone from Copenhagen I very much drew the short straw.

Vinny had to fly straight from Copenhagen to Vienna on business, meaning he was directed to a pleasant and relaxing part of the airport. I, on the other hand, was sent to an area reserved for cattle class in a hangar-like corner of the terminal, made entirely of steel and glass. I nearly fried before being herded on to the plane and focusing on the dubious prospect of collecting our car from Luton Airport's jungle of a car park and driving home in rush-hour traffic via the M1, M25 and M3.

But I got home in one piece while Vinny prepared to run a three-day training course in The Hofburg for a group of senior police officers and administrators from Kyrgyzstan. Despite my hazardous journey, it would be wrong of me to argue that Vinny gets all the best gigs!

My obsession with Hard Rock Cafes has also proved useful on our European travels. During a trip to Croatia, travelling from Split to Dubrovnik via the islands of Hvar and Korčula, we also took the opportunity to take a trip along the Montenegrin coast, dubbed the Russian Riviera due to the many wealthy Russians buying up properties and tracts of land, thereby enabling them to live in style on the doorstep of the EU. We continued to the lakeside town of Kotor, where, tucked away in a corner, we found a tiny Hard Rock Cafe.

Not all our travels abroad have involved flying. For six consecutive years we enjoyed driving to the South of France, where we rented private properties. This choice of destination came about in a rather circuitous manner.

My first diagnosis of cancer in June 2004 came a couple of weeks before the planned trip to Lake Bled in Slovenia, which we had to cancel.

With our replacement holiday in Barbados in January 2005

proving a damp squib (literally), we decided not to book another resort hotel in the summer of that year. We opted instead for a *gîte* and so our sojourns to the South of France began.

Our first trip was to *Pernes-les-Fontaine* in the Vaucluse. I shall never forget the journey down. Having taken the ferry from Dover to Calais and navigated our way round horrendous roadworks on the outskirts of Paris, we stayed overnight at *Mâcon*.

The next morning the sky was leaden-grey, the autoroute was clogged with Parisians heading south and we managed twenty miles in the first hour. I began to wonder whether we had made another huge mistake.

But as we continued, I saw a pinprick of blue just above the horizon. I assured myself that it was not wishful thinking. The further south we drove, the larger it became until we were swathed in a glorious, deep blue *Provençal* sky.

Arrival at our rented villa did not disappoint. It was a typical rustic French property with a large shaded garden and sunlit pool.

Vinny used the word *privacy* to describe that holiday; I used *freedom*. But we meant the same thing – freedom to do as we pleased in the privacy of our own temporary home.

Enjoyable trips out that year included driving across the Camargue to *Aigues-Mortes* and enjoying mango sorbet while admiring the awe-inspiring aqueduct, *Pont du Gard*, near Nîmes.

In *Aigues-Mortes* we did have an amusing parking incident. Even though we arrived early, the limited parking facilities outside the medieval city walls were oversubscribed. We eventually found what we thought was an ideal slot in a long line of parked and unoccupied vehicles near the port area.

We returned several hours later to find our vehicle in

splendid isolation, plastered with very official-looking violation notices and demands. We had evidently parked in a ferry queue, where tradition has it that passengers arrive early to bag a place in line before disappearing for breakfast while awaiting departure time.

We nonchalantly circled the car before jumping in when the coast was clear and beating a hasty (and hopefully inconspicuous) retreat!

Having selected *La Garde-Freinet* in the Var hills, overlooking St Tropez, as the following year's destination, we thought it might be a good idea to let the Motorail take the strain.

How wrong could we be! Not only was the train ancient and the cost exorbitant, there was no restaurant or food of any sort on sale, and only one bathroom per nine compartments, each containing four *couchettes*. I will not trouble you with the state of the ablutions the following morning.

The overall experience was so bad that at the end of the holiday, we opted to drive back instead.

Subsequent years saw us in *Roquebrune-Cap-Martin* in the *Alpes-Maritimes*, from where we could walk into Monaco or drive into Italy; in the Dordogne near Bergerac; and in the *Hautes-Pyrénées* south of Tarbes, where the neighbouring farmer kept geese with *foie gras* tattooed on their foreheads. I can still hear them cackling – briefly!

At another farm across the fields, they served lunch on selected days of the week, created entirely from their own home produce. Wonderful!

Our final trip was to Fitou, way down between Narbonne and

Perpignan in the Aude *département*. It has an unfortunate memory. Lunch on day one knocked Vinny and I out for thirty-six hours with food poisoning. Thankfully, Leah was untouched (a wise choice to have the burger instead of the "fresh" fish).

Our stay coincided with Fitou's annual wine festival. The streets were lined with tables displaying produce from all the local caves. *Vignerons* eagerly provided samples. Unfortunately, Vinny really was not feeling up to it and Leah had yet to acquire the taste. Sampling on my own just was not the same. Such a shame, but I am sure there will be another opportunity.

During those six years we really did explore extensively that whole Mediterranean strip between the Italian and Spanish borders – castles, abbeys, mountain villages, medieval towns *et cetera*. Yet, if you look at a map, we barely touched a fraction of the country as a whole.

Another holiday via boat and car was to the Republic of Ireland. We had a fantastic visit to the west coast in the immediate aftermath of the 2001 foot and mouth fiasco. It was a wonderful holiday, despite the need to wade through various sheep dips on a regular basis. The scenery was magnificent, the weather sympathetic (for Ireland) and the people friendly and hospitable.

It was on this holiday that we renamed lunch as "a fuel stop". We noticed that Leah, who was only four at the time, became very grumpy as lunchtime approached.

Once refuelled, smiles immediately returned, as did her hyper levels of activity. She particularly enjoyed being allowed to sit up at the bar of the local hostelry (Jimmy's) to refuel, as this played well to the rebellious side of her nature.

The holiday stands out for a number of reasons. First, I messed up with regard to half-term dates, resulting in us taking Leah out of school for a week in her first school term. We did not do that again!

Second, the impact of foot and mouth meant not only wading through sheep dips, but also that a crucial Six Nations rugby game between Ireland and England in Dublin had been postponed until our holiday week in October. England lost, and with it the Grand Slam, so we had to endure a great deal of mocking Irish banter.

The third unforgettable element was the journey itself. Starting the holiday with a drive to Swansea, followed by ten hours overnight on the Irish Sea in a tug of a ferry, was perhaps not the best idea. Even those of us with the strongest of sea legs were affected and we all disembarked feeling more than a little queasy. But breakfast at Mother Hubbard's Cafe in Kinsale with the local construction workers soon restored our spirits.

After a drive through the amazing Irish countryside, we arrived in Kenmare. From there we headed out to the Ring of Birra. We took the Ring Road (as opposed to the ring road!) for some distance before turning off on to a single-track road – tarmacked, yes, but with grass growing along the middle. After two miles we arrived at our chosen property.

The cottage was obviously very remote but also very well appointed. Leah immediately took control of the TV and video recorder. Despite having taken a good selection of videos with us, she opted to watch *The Aristocrats* over and over and over again. It is that film that brings back memories of the cottage rather than the accommodation itself or the rural location.

We were generally lucky with the weather, as I have mentioned. It rained overnight but then every morning brought blue sky and sunshine. Obviously, to go out each day, we had to return along the single-track road to the main road. We never saw another vehicle. That was until the day of the most unfortunate aspect of the entire holiday.

Once again it had rained overnight. As we came round a bend we were faced with an approaching vehicle. Vinny pulled into a handy field gate to allow it to pass. As he pulled back out, both front wheels hit wet grass (on the verge and centre of the road), we lost traction, orange lights started to flash on the dashboard, and our heavy car gently rolled into the ditch . . . and refused to budge!

Having extricated ourselves from the situation with no injuries other than to our pride, we realised that we had both left our mobile phones in the cottage. Leaving Vinny with the car, Leah and I walked the mile and a half back to the cottage where I called for assistance.

Some considerable time later, the light flooding into the cottage was suddenly blocked. I looked out of the window to see Vinny clambering down from the largest tractor I have ever seen. The local garage had initially attempted to pull the car out with a 4x4, but ruptured our power steering in the attempt. The garage therefore sought the assistance of a nearby farmer, whose enormous tractor did the trick without any further difficulty. The only damage was to the power steering but, of course, that meant the car was undrivable.

JaguarAssist were marvellous and in no time at all we had a hire car for the rest of the week. (The silver lining was that they also organised a flight home from Cork to Heathrow, where a driver would be waiting for us. Our car would arrive back on a low loader about ten days later for repair at a local garage.)

Our final day was spent enjoying a leisurely stroll around Cork, content in the knowledge that we only had a short flight home to look forward to, rather than another ten hours on the Irish Sea.

Lunch was incredibly pleasant, during which the waitress asked Leah what had been the best moment of her holiday. Leah's response – "When Daddy stuffed the Jag in a ditch!" Out of the mouth of babes!

However, when talking about travel and holidays, one cannot omit the staycation. I do believe that we are truly privileged to live in one of the most beautiful and varied countries in the world, despite having to contend with the vagaries of our weather. We have therefore been at pains to take full advantage of the delights on our doorstep, not least to ensure that Leah developed a balanced appreciation of "home and abroad" as she was growing up.

In addition to driving off for frequent weekend breaks, we have rented cottages at half term in virtually every corner of the UK. In the course of our visits, we have seen a high proportion of what this country has to offer in terms of stately homes, castles (more than Leah cares to remember), churches, cathedrals, homes of the great and good, stone circles, ruins, art galleries and glorious pubs and inns (believe it or not!).

We have also walked countless miles of protected coastline, dales, valleys and woodland (but not peaks!) and visited numerous offshore islands. Our adventures have often taken us off the main tourist track, so Hartlepool features alongside Hardwick Hall and we have been able to compare and contrast Chester with Chester-le-Street!

We have been burned by the sun, soaked to the skin, frozen almost solid and left parched, albeit briefly! We have also stayed in some extremely attractive and quirky properties.

Along the way we have also suffered the odd inconveniences, interruptions and mishaps. On three occasions Vinny was recalled to his office due to unexpected events, for example while in Worcestershire, Derbyshire and the Lake District respectively.

On the first occasion I drove him very early one morning to catch the first train from Worcester Station. In concentrating on the route in an unknown city centre in pre-satnav days, and with no other cars in sight, I was penalised for speeding – thirty-six mph in a thirty mph zone. So, infuriating – particularly given the circumstances.

On the second occasion, Vinny had to return to London for the second half of the week, leaving Leah and me to do our own thing in and around Derbyshire, based in a fantastic upside-down property.

On the third, he managed to restrict his absence to a single day, but that entailed getting the first train out of Oxenholme in the Lake District, and arriving back after midnight – and incurring taxi fares of more than £100 each way!

When Vinny had to leave us in Worcestershire, Leah and I walked across the fields from our splendid cottage to the nearest pub for lunch. The weather turned *en route* and we got soaked. The local farmer drove us home after lunch, which resulted in an invitation to tea the next day with his wife. Well

. . . Leah had tea while the farmer's wife and I cracked open a bottle of wine. Most hospitable!

On arrival at a cottage on the north Northumberland coast, after a long drive, the first thing we discovered at the property was a broken corkscrew. There was only one thing for it. Vinny had to drive the five miles back into Seahouses to acquire a new one. Never again did we go on a cottage holiday without packing a corkscrew and/or a screw-top bottle of wine!

En route to Suffolk, the BMW engine failsafe mode kicked in, resulting in it going into Ipswich for emergency surgery. The courtesy car was a Chevrolet Spark, nothing more than a skip on wheels. Leah leaned against the vehicle, nearly tipping it over.

Vinny suggested, by way of compensation, that we go to watch Ipswich versus Notts County in an FA Cup game at Portman Road. He certainly knows how to make a silk purse out of a hog's ear! I don't know what it is about Notts County, but Vinny also suggested that we go to see them play Carlisle United at Brunton Park on the way back from a holiday in Scotland. Not an experience I would recommend.

The only time we were let down by a property was in Pembrokeshire. We were in an upside-down former watermill in the middle of nowhere. Unfortunately, the property was cramped and damp and the weather was abysmal. We voted with our feet, which included Harvey the dog, and returned home a few days early. The cost of postage to obtain the return of a chunky cardigan left by Leah probably should have been better spent on a new one.

For me, Pembrokeshire was the exception that proves my

rule that cottage holidays are the perfect means to get away, relax and explore. So much better, I believe, to throw things in the back of the car and drive off, than go through the hassle of airport security and so on.

As I write this in the middle of the third Covid-19 lockdown in 2021, we are due imminently to spend two weeks in Wales. For 2022 we already have trips planned to the Scilly Isles and to Orkney and Shetland, two areas of the UK I have always wanted to visit.

A combination of Covid-19 and my cancer diagnosis has obviously forced me to re-evaluate travel which, from a leisure perspective in particular, has given me enormous joy as well as broadening my horizons over a great many years.

Having reflected on past journeys and experiences, and acknowledged how lucky and privileged I have been to venture so far and so often, I have come to the firm conclusion that while I could cope without boarding another flight abroad, I could not live without the opportunity to continue exploring our own green and pleasant land. You just cannot beat it!

14

Art for Art's Sake, Garden for God's Sake

I have always assumed that my love of art was inherited from my mother who, as I mentioned earlier, studied at the Leicester School of Art. I do not claim to have any artistic skills or gifts myself. The only piece of artwork I can remember creating was during my second year at grammar school, or Year Eight as it is now known. As part of the summer examination that year, we were set the task of producing a painting that represented the word *Unity*. I came up with what I thought was a clever idea – a male hand in the act of placing a wedding ring on the ring finger of a female hand.

After a lot of hard work and concentration, I was very pleased with the final outcome until, at the last minute, I realised that the hands were the wrong way round and the painting depicted a left hand putting the ring on to a right hand. No time to make any alterations – I just had to pass it off as a Scandinavian couple.

I would have liked to continue with art despite my limitations, but it was not a feasible option because at that time art was, rather bizarrely, deemed by those in authority within the school to be suitable only for the less academic. Instead, I was forced to choose between German or Physics. Consequently, as with sport, art became more of a spectator interest.

In addition to being members of, and regular visitors to,

the Royal Academy, the Tate, the National Gallery and British Museum, we have invariably created time, and often made significant detours, to track down the less familiar as well as the iconic galleries wherever we have been. There are gems to be found as much in Manchester, Derby, Birmingham or Southampton as in Chicago, Paris, Rome or Vienna.

At the Manchester Art Gallery can be found an excellent collection of paintings by Adolphe Valette, a lesser-known French impressionist painter who greatly influenced his more famous pupil, L.S. Lowry.

Derby Museum and Art Gallery owns the world's largest collection of works by Joseph Wright of Derby. His portrayal of light is quite spectacular.

Birmingham Museum and Art Gallery holds the most important collection of Pre-Raphaelite art anywhere in the world. Southampton City Art Gallery contains work from the Renaissance, through eighteenth- and nineteenth-century British and French art, to a concentration on British twentieth-century and contemporary art.

Although my tastes are quite catholic, I must admit that I am drawn more to Renaissance, Pre-Raphaelite, Impressionist and early twentieth-century modern art than Reformation and extreme modern, such as triptychs and Pollocks!

One of the consequences of all this is that we have managed to collect more art books and paintings or prints than we have shelf or wall space. Vinny's right arm is still longer than his left after carrying two massive volumes of the Thyssen-Bornemisza Collection the two miles from its gallery to our hotel in Madrid.

One tenuous advantage is that we are able to move pictures and prints around when we want a change of scene. But to say we have a repository would be pushing it a bit too far!

After my first bout of cancer in 2004 I was moved to purchase, from a small gallery in Beaulieu, Hampshire, that we visited quite by chance, a glorious painting of children shrimping on a beach. I still regret not buying its accompanying "twin" on the grounds that the cost seemed exorbitant at the time.

As with nature, my present diagnosis has made me appreciate art more keenly and, therefore, during the first Covid-19 lockdown, I embarked on some of the virtual tours and exhibitions that a number of galleries had arranged.

Our magnificent local gallery and framer in Odiham, called simply *The Frame*, had organised a virtual exhibition featuring the internationally renowned wildlife artist Pip McGarry, who has been artist in residence at Marwell Zoo, Hampshire, for twenty years.

When I took a quick look at the review, I fell in love with a limited canvas print, *Leopard in a Tree*, painted from a scene in Botswana. It reminded me of the luck Vinny, Leah and I had in witnessing such a scene, unusual to catch, when we were there in 2013. I therefore had to buy it.

I later had an unexpected, but wonderful conversation with the artist, Pip. Such a charming man. I had a message to call *The Frame* about my purchase and Pip happened to be there. He wanted to know where in Botswana I had taken my own photo of a leopard in a tree (not a patch on his painting!).

That led to discussions about safaris in Botswana. He has been on sixteen, at the time of writing, leading safaris for wildlife artists and photographers. But despite such extensive experience, he was still most interested to hear of our own experience on night-time safaris on the slopes of Chobe, sunset boat-safaris and the infamous mock elephant charge in the Okavango.

He was able to tell me about the Savuti park that runs between Chobe and Okavango (because time constraints dictated that we had flown between the two areas). We then also touched upon safaris in the Masai Mara, Kenya and the Serengeti, Tanzania. We both agreed that the latter were more commercial and Botswana was by far the best.

Such an enjoyable conversation that brought alive so many fortunate and unbelievable memories. He finished off by promising to write a fantastic dedication on the print that I had bought.

The twist in this story is that just after I had determined to purchase the print, I received news from the Department of Work and Pensions that I had been awarded Personal Independence Payment (PIP) with arrears, dating back to March 2000. Although this benefit is paid in recognition of my current immobility and care needs, I am free to use it in any way I see fit to assist with my health and emotional well-being. So what better way to use the arrears than to invest in a print that will bring joy and a smile to my face? The fact that I used PIP to invest in a print by Pip also provided a very neat symmetry!

Despite long experience of viewing great works of art that have been kindly donated or sponsored by wealthy benefactors, I will, however, resist the temptation to add a plate to my Pip McGarry print to the effect that, THE PURCHASE OF THIS PRINT WAS MADE POSSIBLE THROUGH THE KIND GENEROSITY OF THE DWP.

It now sits alongside a second Pip McGarry print of a snow leopard that Vinny kindly bought for my sixtieth birthday.

The Frame gallery has served us well on other occasions. In 2018 my mother turned ninety years of age. The difficult question was what do you give as a present to a ninety-year-old living in a nursing home?

Previously, she had lived in a small village just three miles from us. The average age of the community must be very close to that of my mother, but very active and extremely sociable. With the help of her friends in the village, we gathered together photos of properties and various social gatherings and created a montage. The finished product was expertly framed by the gallery and now hangs on the wall of her room as a lasting memory of her many friends and the fine community spirit they shared over many years.

The Frame also stepped up to the mark when our daughter, Leah, decided that she would like her eighteenth birthday marked not by a wild bash, but by a portrait of her and our dog, Harvey. A suitable artist was sourced by the gallery, who provided the frame, all to stunning effect.

As with live sport, our enjoyment of visiting art galleries has also provided us with many an excuse to travel. For Vinny's fiftieth birthday we spent a long weekend in St Petersburg, home to the magnificent Hermitage Museum, the second largest art gallery in the world.

In addition to the stunning building with its Malachite Room and Main Staircase, its collection of paintings houses works from numerous famous names down through history. We enjoyed an organised guided tour of the highlights, including Michelangelo's *Crouching Boy* and Raphael's *Madonna Contestabile*.

That evening we also enjoyed a culinary delight where the ambience of our chosen restaurant was magical and very reminiscent of the Hermitage. The fare on offer was typically Russian, though served in *nouvelle-cuisine* style. Each meal was accompanied by a complimentary half-bottle of high-quality Russian vodka!

Other lasting memories of this incredible trip included a leisurely stroll around the old markets, a wander down the magnificent Nevsky Prospect and a fascinating visit to the home of poet Alexander Pushkin.

We have also had the good fortune to visit many other European art galleries, including the *Louvre* and *Musée d'Orsay* in Paris, the *Prado* in Madrid, the *Rijksmuseum* and Van Gogh Museum in Amsterdam, the Uffizi in Florence, the Guggenheim in Bilbao, the *Gemäldergalerie* in Berlin, the *Kuntshistoriches* Museum in Vienna and the National Gallery of Ireland in Dublin.

But as I have mentioned, smaller galleries and the homes of the famous – and not so famous – can be just as enjoyable and informative. In Nice, we trudged through the rain to the district of Cimiez where the *Musée Matisse* can be found at the *Villa des Arènes* and which houses one of the world's largest collections of the works of Matisse, one of Vinny's favourite artists.

While in Nice, we also took the opportunity to visit the Renoir and Chagall museums as well as taking a train out to Antibes to explore the *Musée Picasso*.

Another such find is the Rembrandt House Museum in Amsterdam. The interior of the house has been reconstructed to depict how it would have looked in his time and contains a number of his works, as well as those of other Dutch Golden Age painters.

For the summer of 2012 Leah once again selected our choice of holiday destination – a multi-city three-week trip across the northern USA. We flew to Washington D.C., then on to Boston, Cleveland, Chicago and Seattle on internal regional flights before finishing in San Francisco, from where we flew home. I am just so pleased that I was not aware at that time of a National Geographic TV channel programme about air-crash investigations carried out by the US National Transport Safety Board, otherwise I doubt I would have embarked on such an adventure!

Not surprisingly, given the ports of call, we managed to squeeze in a great many visits to some iconic as well as lesser-known art museums during the course of our stay. These included the National Gallery of Art, the Smithsonian American Art Museum and the Hirshhorn Museum and Sculpture Garden in Washington D.C., the Museum of Fine Arts in Boston and the Art Institute of Chicago. These museums feature, along with the Whitney Museum of American Art, the Metropolitan Museum of Art and the Museum of Modern Art in New York, and the Philadelphia Museum of Art – which we have visited on previous trips – in the main top-ten lists of must-visit US art galleries. We really have been incredibly lucky.

One that appears in the *Time* magazine top ten is the Cleveland Museum of Art. Cleveland is not on the main tourist drag and our reason for stopping off there was because friends, Nick and Sue, were living in nearby Chagrin Falls for eighteen months for business reasons. But it did provide Leah with one of the highlights of her trip in that it is home to the *Rock & Roll Hall of Fame.*

In the event, we did not find time to visit the Cleveland Museum of Art, but Vinny harbours more regrets about being unable to visit the Kimbell Art Museum, described as one of the finest in the world, while on a business trip to Fort Worth in Texas.

As in Europe, we found the secondary attractions just as rewarding as their neighbouring A-list sights. For example, The Phillips Collection in the Dupont Circle district of Washington D.C. contains what I consider to be a must-see collection of impressionist art.

Just as beguiling is the Isabella Stewart Gardner Museum in Boston, built and opened by her in 1903 to house her art collection, including works by Vermeer, Titian and Rembrandt, which at the time was regarded as the finest private collection in the world.

While the virtual tours organised by many art galleries during the Covid-19 lockdowns have proved something of a godsend in feeding my culture-vulture tendencies, I cannot wait to get back to viewing fine art from a closer and more intimate perspective. I just hope that when my cancer treatment and the pandemic restrictions ease to allow such a circumstance, constantly peering up from my genetically enforced low-level vantage point will not cause my fractured neck too much discomfort!

As I have mentioned previously, my love of art combines well with that of gardens and gardening, with both being prominent among other passions when I visited Monet's Garden with Vinny for my fortieth birthday. Although I can link my love of art to my mother's chosen pursuit as a student, albeit rather tenuously, I have found it more difficult to trace the source of my horticultural interests. I certainly cannot recall either of my parents being keen gardeners, and neither my sisters nor I really got involved in growing either plants or vegetables. Moreover, I am not sure that I ever saw time spent being creative in the garden as a leisure pursuit of choice until I moved to my current home over thirty years ago.

Looking back, the garden where I now live was a bit of a disaster area when I first moved in, so it is quite possible that necessity triggered my love of gardening and thirst to master the art – or science! I am completely self-taught and realise that the more I learn, the more I do not know, but want to.

One of the first challenges I encountered was not so much about improving the look and feel of the garden, but more in protecting its size from the covetous eyes of the local parish council, who had designs on extending the adjoining church burial ground. *Why us?* I thought. *Why not push back in the opposite direction into the rolling acres of unutilised fields behind? No, let's go for the newbies*, seemed to be the intent.

Appreciating that the inevitable would happen, and considering ourselves fortunate that losing a small part of our land, which could only be used for agricultural purposes, would still leave us with an adequate holding, we entered into discussions with the parish council and its haughty chairwoman.

One morning I was running late for work and happened to notice a mechanical hedge-cutter trundling across our land on its way to cut the adjoining churchyard hedge from our side of the divide.

I shot across our garden and approached the anxious-looking driver.

> Me: "What's going on?"
> Mr Quiver: "She said she'd told everyone."
> Me: "Told? What do you mean, told?"
> Mr Quiver: "I knew there'd be trouble—"
> Me: "Get off my *%^$#!* land!"

I was spitting tacks. The arrogance of it, just to assume that you could, without so much as a by your leave, wander on to someone else's land to carry out a village function.

The exchange was followed by a swift and, I have to admit, somewhat terse missive, reminding the parish council chairwoman that unless and until the land changed hands, she should respect our proprietary rights.

Negotiations ceased, cussedness set in and the parish council were forced down the compulsory purchase route. It did pay off as we got a much better price – and the proceeds were used to buy the TVR D30 vehicle previously mentioned!

So the day came for the completion of the sale and for the new boundary to be delineated. The most unlikely-looking rural district valuer you could imagine attended to do the necessary, dressed in his sharp blue city suit, not a wellie in sight. Still in a cussed state of mind (although I did subsequently mellow and actually served as a parish councillor for four years), I refused to allow the district valuer to cross our land to mark the new boundary and insisted that he enter from the existing churchyard.

At this point the district valuer had not noticed the rams. To keep the grass down, we had two wonderful examples called George and Henry, very affectionate and as docile as you like. I watched with childish amusement as the district valuer, with his borrowed machete, hacked his way through the hedge on to our land. As he came through, he was horror-struck to discover George and Henry were not happy at this intrusion into their world. They had now joined me, waiting close to where the new boundary line would be marked. Their backs came up to my waist (I am only five foot three) and they flanked me on either side, looking like Cerberus and Fang. The three of us stood in a line in stony silence, while the terrified district valuer trembled his way through his tasks, before scuttling off like a petrified dormouse. George and Henry, satisfied with their morning's work, happily returned to their grazing.

Sadly, there came the time when George and Henry had to go to that great abattoir in the sky and they were replaced by a flock of twenty ewes to help keep the grass on the agricultural bit of our land to a manageable level. But they escaped from the field to our adjoining garden with devastating results, including the destruction of my prize giant sunflowers. Consequently, they had to go too. My short-lived days as a shepherdess were over!

Losing part of our field – and the accompanying livestock – meant that I had a little more time to focus on sorting out the garden. I would not claim to be particularly inventive when it comes to garden design and development, so I have tended to look towards the Royal Horticultural Society (RHS) for ideas and inspiration.

I have been a member of the RHS for many years and have always enjoyed visiting their gardens and flower shows. Living within twenty miles of RHS Wisley has made that delightful setting the target for regular visits, come rain or shine. I have also visited RHS Harlow Carr in Harrogate and RHS Hyde Hall near Chelmsford. RHS Rosemoor in Torrington remains on my staycation bucket list.

Over the years we have had many enjoyable visits to the Chelsea Flower Show. The main show gardens have always impressed but my favourites are the smaller, artisan creations. Successful purchases include a courtyard table set, summerhouse and greenhouse.

But there have also been some follies, usually purchased after champagne and sandwiches near the bandstand. Among these ranks a cast-iron crescent-shaped garden seat. Although charming and much improved since Vinny the Restorer wielded his brush and green Hammerite paint during the first Covid-19 lockdown, it is totally impractical. It is nigh on impossible to move and sourcing appropriate-shaped cushions is a non-starter.

Then, of course, there is the must-have, handcrafted Zimbabwean stone bird bath, complete with integral toadstools – I am sure I saw it as a mere snip at the time.

But whether folly or more utilitarian in nature, it is fair to say that all of our Chelsea purchases have stood the test of time . . . but more thanks to being Sourced rather than Made in Chelsea!

One year we took my mother to Chelsea. While on Main

Avenue she became separated from us. I looked around our immediate vicinity and to this day I do not know what she did or how it happened. I tried her mobile phone. No response. We did a circumvention of Main and other avenues and even went to the first-aid tent. I was getting frantic and had that feeling experienced by any parent when losing sight of a child. We are never free of dependents, it would seem – they simply move from one end of the age spectrum to the other in the bat of an eyelid.

I eventually received a call on my mobile from a steward who had found my mother and we were reunited. On enquiring why her mobile was switched off, she cheerfully responded, "I only turn that thing on in emergencies!"

More recently we have been going with friends Nigel and Judy to the members' preview evening at the RHS Hampton Court Flower Show in July. A scrumptious hamper is always provided by Judy as a precursor to a leisurely stroll through the various stands and displays before the evening concludes with a stunning firework display. I have to say that I have come to prefer Hampton Court to Chelsea; there is more room and it feels more relaxed.

There has been much research espousing the benefits of gardening and the outdoor life more generally on our mental health. I certainly recognise those benefits, particularly in relation to the positive psychological effect of witnessing the array of natural colours generated across land, sea and sky as the seasons change.

I recall, in particular, the greatly intensified sense of colour I encountered following my first brush with cancer in

2004. Everything seemed to be presented in high definition compared to my experiences prior to hospitalisation. An autumn visit to the Lake District that year moved me to tears. The following summer, the yellow sunflowers against the deep blue *Provençal* sky was mind-blowing.

That heightened feeling returned with renewed intensity following my second cancer diagnosis in 2020. I wish everyone could experience the same sense of wonderment and joy that is created by seeing things that we often take for granted, such as the force of nature, through a different lens following or during a period of adversity.

That said, I obviously would not want a traumatic event such as a cancer diagnosis to trigger such a reappraisal, but more a non-life-threatening moment on a wander down the road to Damascus.

The timing of my diagnosis in 2020, and the renewed zest for life that it engendered, had the effect of instilling in me an ardent desire to ensure that our garden would look the best and most colourful it has ever been. All I needed to turn my dreams into reality was a fully trained and willing partner in Vinny the Hort!

I launched into my new goal with an unrelenting passion and it was not long before plants and accessories were being delivered, following online purchases, in quantities that Vinny did well to keep track of, let alone under control.

One of the few positive consequences of being housebound due to a combination of chemotherapy treatment and Covid-19 lockdown/shielding, throughout the summer of 2020, was the time and opportunity it created. I ensured that all our pots and hanging baskets were properly watered and that the garden, more generally, was maintained in accordance with a logistical regime that the military would have been proud of.

Often, in previous years, the garden would suffer from holidays taken in July and August, meaning that by September it was already beginning to look sad. The otherwise-to-be-forgotten year of 2020 was very different, with a summer of sustained and glorious colour that lasted until early November. For the first time in many years, I decided to keep all the fuchsias and geraniums and overwinter them in the greenhouse. This involved a useful recycling of some of the cardboard boxes that have arrived as a result of our heavy reliance on online shopping during Covid-19 shielding. Come Spring of 2021, they provided a great start to our creation of a colourful summer and have lasted into the autumn.

My love of gardening has involved growing, or attempting to grow, various vegetables on an almost annual basis, although I am no Monty Don. We have a raised vegetable bed, constructed using old railway sleepers, which is lying dormant at the moment because I have been unable to tend to it with a fractured neck. But it does contain a reasonably sized rhubarb patch, and some asparagus that had been in the ground for four years by spring 2021, so resulting in a decent crop.

With Harvey lodging with friends between April and November of 2020, the local bunnies decided to make hay while the Westie was away. It meant that our garden resembled *Watership Down* at times, and I came to understand why Mr McGregor became so frustrated with Peter Rabbit. Fortunately, a local farmer whose fields surround us decided enough was enough and turned up with his ferrets.

Vinny the Hort undertook a number of garden projects

during the first Covid-19 lockdown in 2020, including the installation of a new bench with planters from where I can enjoy views of the setting sun. More enhanced colour! He appointed me as Assistant Hort and gave me the job of dead-heading all the plants in our pots, over fifty in all.

In previous years I would have regarded this as a necessary chore. But I found the task both enjoyable and cathartic in the wake of time spent recovering from chemo and building up my strength. In the Spring of 2021 I was able to help Vinny plant out all the pots. Small steps forward, but a prelude to progressively bigger and better contributions on the gardening front in future years.

15

Moving On

Life has been a long, joyous and fulfilling journey thus far, with the odd curve ball thrown in. Of the latter, the two marked "cancer" have been particularly unwelcome, but I remain determined to continue batting them away as best I can with the help of my incredible support network, including my family and the incomparable Thin Controller with his highly talented and dedicated team. It would be sacrilege to do otherwise.

As I said to the Thin Controller when he put his black cap on to give me my prognosis, "I have no intention of shuffling off this mortal coil anytime soon." Having slipped past the original six-month sentence, I aim to prolong life for as long as possible and enjoy every additional minute that I am allocated in a spirit of thankfulness and positivity.

With the lyrics of Karen Carpenter's "We've Only Just Begun" ringing in my ears, I decided to embark on the next stage in my life with renewed vigour and optimism. Having, with the help of Vinny and the amazing NHS, navigated my way through a stay in hospital, a grim diagnosis and a rigorous course of intravenous chemotherapy, it was time for me to move on to new horizons.

Yes, I now have incurable metastatic cancer and a related fractured neck that means I must wear a neck brace for life and lose a degree of independence. But that does not mean that a giant full stop has suddenly been inserted in my existence at an inappropriate and untimely juncture; it's more of a semicolon to help me reappraise the direction of travel and make suitable adjustments. Covid-19 obviously had a significant part to play in that mental process if, hopefully, only in the short to medium term.

The first thing I was determined to do, post-intravenous chemotherapy, was to enjoy my sixtieth birthday in August 2020 – the one Leah thought I might just scrape based on my original prognosis!

A repeat of the garden-marquee celebrations that were organised for my fortieth and fiftieth birthdays was clearly out of the question, as was the trip to Tom Kerridge's Michelin-starred *The Hand and Flowers* at Marlow, booked not long before my diagnosis. But we still managed to push the boat out, albeit more in the shape of a canoe than an ocean liner, by hosting Nigel and Judy, along with Leah, for a three-course, socially distanced lunch and bubbles on our courtyard in the late summer sun. Not quite *The Fat Duck* at Bray, perhaps, but for me *The Thin Hogg at Home* was just as innovative and delicious and will live in the memory for as long as the earlier garden parties.

On a more mundane level, an adaptation requiring far less thought was staying slightly longer in bed each morning. The inability to work meant that I no longer needed to rise at the crack of a lark's fart to attend clients finding themselves at their local police station or magistrates' court at short or no notice.

The slight downside to this new-found benefit was being exposed for a little longer to the ramblings and rantings of those who do combat each morning on BBC Radio 4's *Today* programme. The voices of James Naughtie, John Humphrys and Sue MacGregor *et al* have for many years been the first Vinny and I hear in the morning as our audio-alarm signals the start of another working day. It is a habit that we found almost impossible to break, despite the sharp diminution in the quality and influence of the programme in recent years.

However, we did eventually jump ship in the summer of 2020 and now wake up to the dulcet tones of Steve Allen and Nick Ferrari on LBC.

The catalyst for this change was the increasingly negative slant that the Today programme was placing on the majority of news items emerging during the early days of the pandemic, combined with a tendency to be less focussed on detail and accuracy. A prime example concerned the adverse impact that a stretched NHS was said to be having on the treatment of cancer patients. The picture presented was so critical, and far removed from my own positive experience, that I felt compelled to email a complaint to the BBC. Needless to say I did not receive the courtesy of a reply.

Just before switching my allegiance to LBC, the *Today* programme, in referring to people like myself who would need to continue to 'shield' in self-isolation regardless of whatever imminent steps might then be taken to ease the Covid-19 lockdown restrictions, mentioned an NHS letter that it reported had been sent to everyone in my situation. The letter, it was said, explained why our vulnerability demanded self-isolation, and provided an evidential basis for access to special support services, such as supermarket deliveries.

The radio feature reminded me that I, and many others in a similar position, had still not received such a letter due to a major administrative glitch that had not been made public, but was explained to me by my local GP surgery. This despite emailing my MP, who had cited the existence of such a letter in trumpeting the alleged success of government Covid-19 policy some weeks previously, an email that remains unanswered to this day.

Fortunately the absence of the NHS letter had little impact at a practical level. This was largely because we have acquired a fairly good understanding of how public sector systems and processes work and, with a few exceptions, how best to proceed when these break down.

Consequently, the extra work involved in organising preferential services, such as supermarket deliveries, without NHS evidence presented no more than a minor irritant. However, I do feel very sorry for those who are understandably intimidated and frustrated by bureaucracy, especially when operatives at the end of the telephone line lack the time and discretion to find practical solutions, often resorting to the default position of overpromising but under-delivering, on the basis of rigid, but deficient, corporate guidelines and processes.

However, this experience of securing preferential treatment from the likes of Sainsbury's proved invaluable in retrospect. This was because my more limited independence and mobility meant that even after the lifting of lockdown restrictions, I would have to rely much more heavily on online shopping and forgo the delights of regular trips to the local high street or Westfield-type horror shows.

I say this slightly tongue-in-cheek because, despite my pathological loathing of any form of shopping, I have tended to make the physical journey rather than bash the keyboard, partly out of habit, and partly out of the perceived unreliability of online service delivery. In other words, a fear – justified to a certain extent on early experience – that the right goods will not turn up at the right place at the right time, and that the wrong amount will be debited from my account. Moreover, that none of the failings would be capable of being resolved because of the Kafkaesque nature of the corporate entities supplying the various goods and services involved.

But my inability to just jump in the car and drive to the shops as the need arose, both short and long term, meant that I would need to embrace online shopping and put my concerns, whether justified or irrational, to one side.

I nevertheless anticipated that increasing my reliance on online shopping from around fifteen per cent to one hundred per cent might prove particularly troublesome, coming as it did at a time when home deliveries were rising exponentially due to lockdown restrictions. I was not disappointed!

I must admit that I stepped rather gingerly into the online fray after leaving hospital in late March 2020. Having eventually ensured that all the regular essentials of life would be delivered through Sainsbury's, I became less concerned about ordering what I would regard as luxuries, or at least items that are not entirely necessary to keep me alive and functioning.

Into the latter category fell some lightweight scarves that I selected to cover my neck brace, not because I am embarrassed about wearing it, but more to alleviate the discomfort that some people clearly encounter in trying to avoid looking at it. Other online purchases included clothing to suit my new circumstances (eg replacing tops, such as T shirts, that are tight around the neck), various items designed to improve the appearance of the garden (eg plants, pots and trellis), kitchen tools and gadgets, and the occasional folly aimed largely at helping to support small businesses during lockdown.

The associated delivery experiences included parcels being left hidden under our front hedge or in diverse locations around the village, attempted illegal forced entry to obtain signatures, despite medical shielding notices on doors and windows (enter Vinny the Protector to "have a word"), drivers phoning (or giving up) after landing in a completely different village or postcode, and consignments destined for other properties, far and wide, being left clandestinely on various parts of our property, presumably in desperation.

Despite these experiences, we have been able to make the total reliance on online shopping work, thanks mainly to the use of social media and the kindness and cooperation of friends and neighbours. Moreover, the inconvenience caused has not been in the same league as that encountered on occasions prior to the Covid pandemic. Two historic instances spring readily to mind.

On the first such occasion we were forced into making an unusual complaint when a courier left a trampoline cover that we had ordered at the rear of the neighbouring property and took delight in urinating against the back door in the process. The company's curious attempt at restitution was to send another trampoline cover!

On the second occasion, a courier dropped a box over our garden gate one Christmas Eve when Vinny was standing close by. Unfortunately, the courier was extremely quick in making his getaway because the parcel was not for us but for someone in the village whose name and (incomplete) address we did not recognise. We did, however, manage to track down the rightful owners after much detective work, who were extremely grateful as the parcel contained their Christmas turkey!

On balance, and despite the types of issue I have highlighted, I have gradually become accustomed to the life of an exclusive online shopper and all the associated problems that can occur, particularly with regard to deliveries.

As with most irritants in life, the occasional frustrations arising from the vagaries of online deliveries erode quite sharply when viewed with a degree of inevitability and acceptance, and I have to say that being able to shop from the sofa beats wandering around the average shopping mall hands down.

Adjusting to reliance on the internet for all of my shopping needs proved quite straightforward from a mental-acceptance perspective compared to another change necessitated by my medical circumstances. I'm referring to the transition from full-time employment to applying for benefits to which I had suddenly become entitled.

I have been in some form of gainful employment since the age of eleven, and it was indoctrinated in me from that early age that one had to be financially self-sufficient throughout one's life. The idea of not being able to support oneself through initiative and hard work, and turning to the State for help, were a complete anathema. The idea of no longer being able to earn an income through the application of the professional skills I had developed and cherished, and instead have to apply for financial entitlements to the Department for Work and Pensions (DWP), was one of the cancer-inducing life changes that I found the most difficult to accept.

It took some prodding and persuasion from my magnificent Macmillan nurses before I became reconciled with the fact that I was entitled to financial support from the State and should therefore make the appropriate application.

In addition to describing the principal entitlement appropriate to my circumstances, the Macmillan nurses explained the processes that apply, including the fast-track systems that are in place for those with Stage 4 cancer.

I soon discovered that theory and practice are not always closely aligned when it comes to applications for financial benefits. However, with Vinny's help, I managed to successfully navigate the fast-track system and, as a result, it was not long before a weekly benefit in the form of a Personal Independent Payment (PIP) was hitting my bank account.

Having cleared the necessary hurdles to reach this particular point, the Macmillan nurses then suggested that I might also be eligible for the new-style Employment and Support Allowance (ESA). I therefore did the appropriate homework before lodging an application, but this time hit more of a barrier with that part (or, more accurately, those parts) of the DWP who deal with such claims.

The impression I'd gained as a result of the problems encountered with my PIP application was that they were due to dysfunctional DWP systems and processes, which perseverance on my part would eventually overcome. However, there seemed to be more of a systematic attempt to put ESA claimants off persisting with their claims by placing different obstacles in their path at regular intervals, while simultaneously complicating the bureaucracy on an incremental basis.

By way of example, I was initially advised by the DWP that I was not eligible for new-style ESA payments because, in two relevant years, I had not paid sufficient National Insurance Contributions (NICs). However, because of my medical position, I would nevertheless be credited with ongoing NICs.

I was subsequently informed that the NIC credits would cease because Covid-19 shielding was nearing its conclusion. When I pointed out that my ESA application was made on the basis of my medical situation and was not Covid-19 related, I was told my claim would be reopened.

Not long after that I was informed that the previous adviser had "misspoken" and that I would have to resubmit my application. I therefore made good the missing NICs and duly reapplied.

The next communication I received from the DWP was to advise that my application had not been successful because my NICs were not up to date, despite having made the appropriate payment to fill the gap!

I remained in regular touch with the DWP about my application and each time felt that the operative I was speaking to was starting afresh, with no progress having been made in between. On one occasion, during a call lasting over one hour, I was given conflicting information about the state of play because of internal confusion as to the status of the claim and, therefore, which office in the UK might be dealing with it.

My plea that I would welcome due priority being assigned to my claim because time is running out and, according to my initial prognosis, I should already be dead, did not seem to cut any ice.

Once again a request for assistance from my MP proved fruitless in that his referral to the DWP did not elicit a response and has not been followed up almost a year later. Having, meanwhile, identified a potential resolution, and written to the HMRC accordingly, my letter remains unanswered three months later.

I mention my post-diagnosis foray into the mysterious and previously unexplored world of benefits at some length because it has proved a rather daunting and frustrating experience. I am fortunate that I have the time and patience (just) to deal with the complex bureaucracy and knock-backs involved, and that whether I eat or where I sleep is not dependent on the nature and speed of the DWP or HMRC responses. My heart goes out to those less fortunate than myself who have to deal with the systems and processes involved without the same levels of experience, resource and resilience.

Looking at the benefits, in the widest sense of the word, of being a long-term cancer patient with a fractured neck, one tangible perk that readily springs to mind is the entitlement to a Blue Badge for disabled persons.

This might sound like a rather odd *plus* to cite, particularly as I love driving and have had to come to terms with the probability that my neck brace is for life unless, through some miracle, corrective neck surgery proves possible and is sufficiently successful to give me the manoeuvrability to sit behind the wheel again. But as with all the post-diagnosis adjustments I have had to make, I tend to focus on the pro side of the balance sheet and dismiss, or at least moderate, the cons.

On a similar basis, Vinny the Chauffeur has argued that the disappointment of no longer being able to share the joy of driving on long journeys will be counterbalanced by the ability to sneak into a disabled space in crowded car parks rather than drive around willing people to leave as stress levels increase.

He also took the opportunity for some light-hearted payback by reminding me how I had laughed when, on the day some years ago, I took possession of a mid-life crisis Mercedes SLK, he received an unsolicited motor insurance quote for those aged over 50 from Saga!

There was not much opportunity to test out the Blue Badge during Covid-19 lockdowns one and two. There were a few disabled spaces at the Shunting Shed, when based on the Island of Sodor, for us to sample. When we had to go to Mainland and park outside the front door, Jobsworth the Security Guard was unable to bark at me as he is wont to do.

I am sure a Blue Badge Society must exist that, rather like the Ramblers, runs trips out on a Sunday. But if there is, I will probably give it a miss.

When the Blue Badge arrived, it came in two parts – the badge itself and a circular card clock used to indicate time of arrival in a parking space. I decided it would be useful to order a suitable cover from Amazon to hold the two parts for easy display on the dashboard.

Shortly after receipt of my order, I received an email from Amazon about "a recommendation based on a recent purchase". The recommended item was described thus . . .

- *Don't Get Caught Without One of these Perfect Time Savers!*
- *Must-have for Disabled Access to Locked Public Facilities!*

What was the item? A Disabled Toilet Radar Key! The things I am learning in my brave new world!

I am hoping that in addition to the obvious benefits, the presence of a Blue Badge on the dashboard will help avoid parking issues similar to those experienced in the past.

Once, while building works were taking place at HMP Winchester, parking was a bit of a free-for-all. Squeezing into the last available space, I accidentally reversed over a six-inch parapet. No damage was done but the car was immobile. Fortunately, a couple of lads nearby had spotted my predicament and immediately lifted my car back on to the driveway. How embarrassing, but I was extremely grateful for prison trusties performing external tasks!

Perhaps the most entertaining parking issue of all occurred on our own drive. A friend brought to our attention serious talk in the village that our marriage might be in difficulties. The reason for this show of concern? It had been noticed that the gap between our parked cars on the drive was growing wider!

I have to admit I find it odd to think of myself as registered disabled. I may not be able to drive, my neck is supported by braces Nefie or Stretch and, when I go out wrapped in one of my scarves, I look like a guerilla or a bank robber. But I still call out the answers when watching *Pointless* on TV, still shout at the contestants on *Eggheads* when they choose to go second, or at the contestants on *Who Wants to Be A Millionaire?* when they waste a lifeline, and I still love sport and hate shopping (even when it is out of bounds). In my head, I am still ever the same.

Having reflected on the term *disabled*, following

confirmation of my entitlement to benefits and a Blue Badge, I decided to do some research.

Oh dear. What a politically correct minefield the world of disability is. This does not bode well for someone such as me who has to contend, on a daily basis, with an overload of gallows humour.

There is plenty of advice on words *not* to use, such as *spastic, retarded, crippled* and *handicapped*. Even *physically challenged* is unacceptable to some because it places emphasis on an individual's disabilities as opposed to their abilities. In fact, you should not even concentrate on abilities but on the person as a whole. Hence the most appropriate term, evidently, is *person with disability*, although *disabled* is a perfectly acceptable alternative. Or so they say!!

Quite frankly, I cannot see what is wrong with the term *physically challenged*. There are a number of physical activities that I presently find challenging but I do not think of myself as disabled. I appreciate that disabled persons have rights and I would never use a term in relation to others that may cause offence in any way. However, I have rights too, which include allowing me to refer to myself as *physically challenged* should I choose to do so. That being said, I certainly do not want to fall foul of the disability PC *Gauleiters*, so I have decided to devise my own individualised term.

My physical challenges stem almost entirely from having to wear a neck brace. Mobility has improved considerably in that I can now negotiate the stairs normally – as opposed to one step at a time when I first came out of hospital; I can put on my own socks; and I can go for long walks. But I will not be looking back over my shoulder, physically or metaphorically, anytime soon and I have cancelled my gym membership. So I am not alone in this Covid-19 dominated world in having to adapt to a new normal way of operating.

In looking for an alternative to *disabled* to describe my new situation, I came across the word *isometric*. Having determined, from the derivation and meaning of the word, that I remain essentially isometric, and having taken account of the PC *Gauleiters'* diktat regarding individualism, I have decided that the term that best describes my physical condition is *issyometric*!

Returning to my balance sheet of driving disability pros and cons, one of the benefits I placed on the pro side was the fact that I would never be stopped by the police again. I should begin here by stating, in my defence, that I have not had regular interaction with those of our policing friends assigned to road-traffic duties. But on the few occasions that I have, my policy has always been to be positive and proactive.

While on holiday in Aldeborough, Suffolk, Vinny and I were stopped by a Police Community Support Officer (PCSO) for speeding. He approached and spoke to Vinny through his window.

PCSO Insufferable: "Do you realise you were speeding?"

Vinny: "I'm terribly sorry. I thought we had already left the thirty mph limit."

PCSO Insufferable: "Do you realise how dangerous it is to speed? Even at lower speeds fatal injuries can be caused. You're not local. I don't want to see tourists tearing around on our roads. You're very lucky that today we are giving verbal warnings and not issuing tickets."

Me: (staring out of my window, biting my tongue as hard as possible to prevent myself blurting out to PCSO Insufferable that PCSOs did not, at that time, have the power to issue tickets!)

Vinny: (also aware of the lack of power) "Thank you, Officer. Most kind."

We drove on, discretion being the better part of valour.

When I was six months pregnant with Leah, I was so huge that I could not comfortably get the seatbelt round my midriff. While driving in Basingstoke, a police car suddenly appeared behind me and motioned me to stop.

PC Assiduous: "Do you know why I've stopped you?"

Me: "Yes, Officer. I'm afraid I can't get the seatbelt round me but, no, I don't have a certificate from my doctor."

PC Assiduous: "Aren't you a solicitor in Farnborough?"

My heart sank. But fortunately, and despite recognising me, he allowed me on my way with a direction to get a certificate from the doctor exempting me from the requirement to wear a seatbelt.

On another occasion in Basingstoke, a police car pulled out rapidly behind me. I was wearing a baseball cap over short hair (therefore from a distance perhaps appearing masculine) and driving a BMW. I knew I was going to be stopped and sure enough, a few seconds later, it was nee-naw time. As the officer approached my window, he said . . .

PC Fluster: "Good afternoon, sir."

> Me: (turning towards him, smiling sweetly and handing him my driving licence) "Good afternoon, Officer."
>
> PC Fluster: (stumbling over his words) "Oh, oh, sorry, madam. Er, um, we've had a number of high-value car thefts . . ."
>
> Me: "I can assure you I'm not a car thief."
>
> PC Fluster: "No, no, of course. Sorry, madam. Please carry on."

My love of driving before my diagnosis was matched, and probably exceeded by, my love of cooking. But whereas I found ways of being able to put my driving days behind me, that was never going to be possible with life in the kitchen.

When I first came out of hospital, there was little that I could do on the meal-preparation front, which I found most frustrating because of the joy I have always derived from cooking and the extent to which the kitchen has been my domain.

But Vinny the Pinny more than stepped up to the plate. Throughout the weeks and months that followed, he continued to produce some excellent home-made soups and now creates them without reference to recipes.

We gradually moved from the strange sight of Vinny dominating the kitchen, to me preparing a simple main element to which he added the accompaniment, for example, his broccoli tossed in rapeseed oil, rice wine and crushed garlic, dusted with grated Parmesan, then roasted to complement my pork medallions; or his green lentil, celery and mushroom side dish to my chicken Milanese.

Over time I got back to cooking complete meals and, while still shielding, we had friends for socially distanced alfresco lunches when the weather allowed, assisted by patio heaters.

But Vinny still provides assistance in the kitchen with preparation. I rather like it because he creates a mini version of BBC's *Saturday Kitchen* by preparing all the ingredients and placing them in individual bowls ready for me to use.

Vinny has never really trusted me with sharp knives, which partly explains the reason for this new *modus operandi*. My vulnerability has simply given him the excuse to remove all sharp objects from my reach.

Early on in my chemo treatment, I was getting to that irritating stage of wanting to contribute more in the kitchen. I offered, for example, to peel and chop the vegetables. Vinny's response – "No way – you were a bloody nuisance with sharp kitchen utensils before this!"

I was reminded of an incident about twenty years ago. While preparing lunch one Saturday I managed to slice my left index finger halfway to the bone! "You stupid woman!" I heard him mutter, though like Jeremy Corbyn and John Bercow more recently, he now denies saying it. The trouble was that England were about to open their televised Six Nations rugby campaign and neither of us fancied an afternoon in A&E. Vinny bound it up really tightly for the weekend.

After being first on in Aldershot Magistrates' Court on the Monday, I toddled off to A&E. It was too late to stitch the wound but what a marvellous job Vinny had done. I still struggle even now to find the scar.

The reminder of this incident was Vinny's way of rebuffing my offer of help, and he has remained firmly in charge of the kitchen knives! But I am rather pleased with myself that I have managed to inveigle my way back into the kitchen and am enjoying cooking as much as I did before cancer rudely intervened.

Travel and live sport also offer a realistic prospect of returning to new-normal life in a post Covid-19 world, albeit on a more limited scale than has proved possible in the past. In common with most other interests, hobbies and functions post-diagnosis, I have come to terms with the fact that I will have to lower my horizons somewhat. For example, long-haul travel will clearly be off the agenda, while attendance at major sporting events will require a degree of risk management.

But my analysis of what may or may not be possible has again revealed plenty of exciting opportunities and possibilities, with a strong focus on staycations – and even some short-haul foreign trips. With some innovative thinking and planning, I am confident that I can reach my slightly revised goal of visiting sixty countries before I reach the age of sixty-two, with my sights set firmly on Norway (a two-week cruise around the fjords having already been booked for June 2022), Switzerland and Liechtenstein as the three countries needed to reach my target.

The absence of live spectator sport left a large gap in my life after my diagnosis, but the concurrence of Covid-19 and related restrictions meant that attendance at sporting events would not have been possible in any case. However the easing of restrictions has meant returning to the Ageas Bowl in Southampton to watch cricket. Spectators are very well spaced around the ground and masks must still be worn when walking around away from your seats.

On a brighter note, we were able to change the seats covered by our Bath Rugby season tickets at the Recreation Ground to a location that is far more comfortable for me and easier to access. Once again the club were absolutely stunning in the assistance that they provided to accommodate my change in circumstances. The new season started in September 2021 and the new seats lived up to expectation.

Inevitably, the risks of attending major sporting events are more difficult to predict so we will need to assess those on a case-by-case basis. The same is true of other events attracting large crowds, such as popular art exhibitions and central London theatres, but I am not prepared to rule anything out without drawing up a list of pros and cons and assessing the risks.

I have no doubt that there will be further twists and turns along the path ahead, and that I will need to make additional adjustments to the way I live my life as time goes by. But life is not an entitlement, more a sacred and wonderful gift, as my memories have testified, so I have every intention of turning any fresh challenge I face into another new opportunity.

It is an oft-quoted truism that those who are nearest and dearest are impacted just as severely, if not more so, when a family member or close friend is faced with a life-threatening or changing situation. I therefore owe it to them, as much as to myself, to continue to approach life in the same positive frame of mind so that we are able to share the rewards of such positivity to the same extent in the future as we have in the past. I also hope that my continued zest for life, and refusal to be beaten, will in some small and humble way prove inspirational to others beyond my circle of family and friends, whatever challenges they may face.

Life is just so glorious and I cannot wait to begin the next chapter.

Carpe diem!

Epilogue

As I stood on the Pembrokeshire Coastal Path admiring the stunning scenery of St Brides Bay (*basophobia* be damned!) while on our summer 2021 staycation, I reflected on the fifteen months since my initial cancer diagnosis. It was a happy rather than sad reflection, not least for having enjoyed life for nine months longer than the medics originally predicted. And I was still counting!

I have successfully navigated my way through six cycles of chemotherapy and my cancer has been stable since September 2020 thanks to the oral medication I am now on. Moreover, the results of my latest CT scan in October 2021, given to me by Chief Engineer Empathy, revealed a significant shrinkage in the lesions on my liver. Our conversation was remarkably calm despite the Cornish pixies and mischievous elves deciding it was time for an impromptu party in my mental office!

Vinny and I have cheerfully survived over a year of extreme shielding. The particular joy of emerging from this situation was the ability to have a family hug with Leah after fourteen months of no physical contact. She has found new accommodation and a rewarding job that she thoroughly enjoys.

On one recent occasion I was, at last, able to visit my mother and, despite her dementia, she recognised us instantly – although she was somewhat shocked to see Vinny, having convinced herself that he had died two days previously. The one blessing of her condition is that she has no concept of time, so has no idea of the length of time since she last saw us

– and remains unaware of my situation. On medical advice I will continue visits remotely for now (ie through video) while the Covid risks remain given my supressed immune system.

I have become a bit racy – well, for me anyway. I now sport purple hair and glasses very much in the spirit of the wonderful 1961 poem by Jenny Joseph, *Warning*, better known by its first line, "*When I Am an Old Woman I Shall Wear Purple . . .*"

Sadly, my middle sister, Kate, has been diagnosed with pancreatic cancer. But she is as upbeat as me and continues to work. I, on the other hand, have decided to hang up my wig and gown on medical grounds and enjoy a well-earned retirement after thirty-seven years of legal cut and thrust. However, I will retain my practicing certificate - just in case!

On a wall in St David's Cathedral in Pembrokeshire, I noticed the following words – "*What scars do you carry, physical or mental? Can you see in them your ability to survive what life throws at you?*" I was immediately reminded of the lyrics of one of my favourite songs, Gloria Gaynor's "I Will Survive". If you think of cancer as the spurned lover, the words are spot on.

I will survive!!

October 2021